GYMNASTIC ACTIVITIES • DANCE • GAMES

PE LESSON PLANS

year 2

COMPLETE TEACHING PROGRAMME

WITHDRAWN

SECOND EDITION

LEAPFROGS

JIM H

A music CD with tracks to accompany many of the Dance lessons in this series is available separately (ISBN: 978 07136 7902 1).

Relevant tracks are indicated on each lesson page with the following logo:

Published in 2009 by A & C Black Publishers Ltd,
an imprint of Bloomsbury Publishing Plc
50 Bedford Square, London, WC1B 3DP
www.bloomsbury.com

Reprinted 2012
Copyright © 2009 by Jim Hall

ISBN 978 14081 0995 3

A CIP record for this book is available from the British Library.

Note: While every effort has been made to ensure that the content of this book is as technically accurate and as sound as possible, neither the author nor the publisher can accept responsibility for any injury or loss sustained as a result of the use of this material.

A & C Black uses paper produced with elemental chlorine-free pulp, harvested from managed sustainable forests.

Acknowledgements
Cover illustration by Tom Croft
Cover design by James Watson
Illustrations by Jan Smith

Typeset in 10pt DIN Regular.

Printed and bound in Croatia by Zrinski.

Contents

Introduction

Because an increasing number of young children today do not have the opportunity to take part in regular play, physical activity or exercise, enjoyable, vigorous, well taught physical education lessons are more important than ever. Equally important is a sense of staff unity regarding the 'Why?', the 'What?', and the 'How?' of physical education to deliver a whole school, successful programme with continuity and high standards from year to year. The main reasons for teaching physical education, include:

Physical development: First and foremost, the main reason for teaching physical education has always been to inspire vigorous, enjoyable, challenging and wholehearted physical activity that develops normal healthy growth and satisfactory development of each pupil's strength, suppleness and stamina. The skills taught also aim to develop skilful, confident, well-controlled and safe movement. It is hoped that the varied skills will give pleasure and satisfaction, catering for many interests and aptitudes, and will eventually enable pupils to take part in healthy, worthwhile and sociable activities long after they have left school. These skills, learned and enjoyed at school, are remembered by the body for a very long time.

Personal, social and emotional development, compensating for the near total disappearance of play in the out-of-school lives of many of our pupils. It is reported that millions of children spend most of their free time – up to five hours every day – watching a TV or a computer screen. It has also been claimed that parents, who refuse to let their children go out to play, are producing a 'battery-farmed' generation who will never become resilient and will be unable to deal with risk.

This lack of play means no exercise, no fresh air, no physical development, no social development though interaction with others, no adventure in challenging situations and no emotional development. It has been said 'an individual's regard for, and attitude to, his or her physical self, especially at primary school age, is important to the development of self-image and the value given to self.' Physical education lessons are extremely visual, providing many opportunities for demonstrating success, creativity, versatility and enthusiastic performances which should be recognised by the teacher, praised and commented upon, and shared with others who should be encouraged to be warm in their praise and comments. Such successes can enhance a pupil's feelings of pride and self-confidence.

The play-like nature of physical education lessons is obvious. In games, running, jumping and landing, throwing and catching, batting, skipping, trying to score points or goals; in gymnastic activities, running, jumping and landing, rolling, climbing, swinging on ropes, balancing, circling on bars; and in dance, skipping, running and jumping, travelling with a partner, a group or a circle in performing a dance, are all playful actions in which pupils find fun and satisfaction from performing well, and social development from being in the company of others.

When teaching physical education lessons now, teachers need to remember that the lessons may be providing the only active play that some of the pupils will experience that week. The lessons must be vigorous, enjoyable, and give an impression of children at play.

Contributing to pupils' health now, and long after they have left school. The health of our children and eventually the health of our nation, has been a cause for concern for university researchers and health experts for decades. A 1997 headline described British children as 'The Flab Generation'. It was estimated in 2000, that in a class of thirty children, two will go on to have a heart attack, three will develop diabetes, and thirteen will become obese, all as result of a sedentary lifestyle and a diet dominated by chips, biscuits, sweets and sugary drinks. A 2002 report revealed that a third of 10 year olds did not even walk continuously for ten minutes a week.

The above statistics and figures have become far worse since those early ignored warnings. The NHS treated 85,000 patients for clinical obesity in 2007 and it is estimated that by 2020, 50% of all children in Britain will be obese. England has the fastest growing weight problem in Europe. The link between obesity and diabetes is well known and 100,000 UK patients are diagnosed with type 2 diabetes every year, fuelled by the nation's obesity problem. Douglas Smallwood, Chief Executive of the charity Diabetes UK says 'Diabetes is a serious condition which can lead to devastating complications such as blindness, amputation, heart and kidney disease.' Almost one hundred diabetics a week have a limb amputated because of complications with their disease.

An extra twelve kilograms in weight boosts the risk of cancer by 50%. Coronary heart disease causes 105,000 deaths a year and 2.6 million people are thought to be living with the symptoms of heart disease. Scientists have warned that unfit, lazy children are six times more likely to develop early signs of heart disease than those who are active and take exercise. For the first time, experts have established that activity levels in children as young as seven can have a serious effect on their future health. Professor Paul Gately, of Leeds Metropolitan University says 'Inactive children at a relatively young age are already storing up health risks for the future.' Health specialists, concerned for the health of our nation, are now repeatedly emphasising the importance of regular exercise as the best way to reduce the risks of suffering life-threatening illnesses in later life.

The National Obesity Forum has called for urgent action to tackle the obesity problem which, they calculate, causes 30,000 deaths each year and emphasises that the time to act is in childhood before irreversible damage has been done, and while lifelong habits can be learned. British Heart Foundation research found that taking 30 minutes of moderate exercise most days reduces the risk of an early death by more than a quarter. Diabetes UK warns that obesity is making a diabetes epidemic inevitable. Physical activity and a sensible diet are the best ways to reduce the risk of developing diabetes. The World Cancer Research Fund 2007 Report, produced by scientists and medical experts from around the world, tells us that most cancers are preventable by choosing a healthy diet, being physically active and maintaining a healthy weight. They recommend being physically active for at least 30 minutes every day, to keep the heart healthy and to reduce the risk of cancer.

Realistically, it is only in schools in physical education lessons, that we can encourage and help children to succeed in a wide range of physical skills and inspire, motivate and facilitate a joy in physical activity that will combat the health problems mentioned above. Physical education makes a unique contribution to an all-round, balanced education, but it also makes a special contribution to a life-prolonging, healthy lifestyle. For today's primary school children regular, excellent, vigorous and enjoyable physical education lessons are probably the best health products they will ever receive.

Teaching Physical Education

The teacher of physical education, almost uniquely, works alone and unaided, and is involved in whole class teaching with no help from the mass of teaching aids that help to keep pupils purposefully and often independently engaged in their classrooms. Even if he or she is talking to an individual, a pair or a small group, the teacher in a physical education lesson still needs to be aware of the whole class and how it is responding to the set task.

The teacher is the source and inspiration for everything that happens in the lessons. He or she needs to be well prepared to make the lesson complete, enjoyable, stimulating and challenging; enthusiastic to create an equally enthusiastic response; warm and encouraging to help pupils feel pleased and good about themselves; and intensely interested in inspiring vigorous physical activity in pupils, many of whom, away from school, may have inactive and sedentary lifestyles.

The lesson plan is the teacher's essential guide and reminder of the current lesson's content. Failure to plan and record lessons results in the same or similar things being done, month after month. Parts of the lesson gradually disappear, and an unprepared teacher can finish up doing no teaching in a lesson where everything is vague or has been done before. Pupils at apparatus in such an unprepared lesson answer 'Nothing' when asked 'What has your group been asked to do at this apparatus?'

July's lesson will only be at a more advanced stage that the previous September's if all the lessons in between have been recorded and referred to, to make each succeeding lesson move on and introduce new, interesting and exciting challenges. The lesson usually runs for four or five weeks (one lesson per week) to give the class enough time to practise, improve, develop, learn, remember and enjoy all the skills involved.

'Dead spots' and queue avoidance. The 'scenes of busy activity' which every physical education lesson should be requires an understanding by all pupils that they should be 'found working, not waiting'. This means that they need to be trained to respond immediately, behave well, keep on practising until stopped, and avoid standing immobile in queues.

The teacher needs to avoid talking the class out of their lesson through over-long explanations, demonstrations and pupil reflections following demonstrations. Lessons that lose a lot of time result in unsatisfactory, hurried apparatus work, frustratingly short time for playing games, and half-created dances with no time to share them proudly, with the class.

Demonstrations and observations by pupils and teacher are essential teaching aids because we remember what we see – good quality work; safe, correct ways to perform; the exact meanings of physical education terminology; and good examples of variety and interesting contrasts. All can watch one, two or a small group. Half of the class can watch the other half. Each can watch a partner. These occasional demonstrations, with comments by the observing pupils, often bring out good points not noticed by the teacher; train pupils to understand the elements of 'movement'; and let teachers ask 'how can it be improved?' Making friendly, encouraging, helpful points to classmates is good for class morale and for extending the class repertoire in physical education. ('Occasional' means once or twice at most in one lesson because of the time taken to do this.)

Further class practice should always follow a demonstration so that everyone can try to include some of the good features praised and commented on.

Shared choice or **indirect teaching** takes place when the teacher decides the nature of the activity and challenges the class to decide on the actions. Limits set are determined by the experience of the pupils. From the simple 'Can you travel on the apparatus, using your hands and feet?' with its slight limitations, we can progress on to 'Can you travel on the apparatus, using hands and feet, and include a still balance, a direction change, and taking all the weight on your hands at some point?'

Shared choice teaching produces a wide variety of results to add to the class repertoire. Being creative is extremely satisfying and most primary school pupils enjoy and are capable of making individual responses.

Direct teaching takes place when the teacher tells the class what to do, including, for example: any of the traditional gymnastic skills; the way to hold, throw and catch a ball; or how to do a folk dance step. Correct, safe ways to move; support yourself; grip, lift and carry apparatus; and throw implements, are all directly taught.

If the class is restless, not responding, or doing poor work, a directed activity can restore interest and discipline and provide ideas and a valuable starting point from which to develop. Pupils who are less interested, less inventive or less gifted physically, will benefit from direct teaching, particularly if the teacher can suggest an alternative, simpler but equally acceptable idea. 'If you do not like rolling forwards, try rolling sideways instead. Start, curled up on your back, with your hands clasped under your knees. This keeps your head out of the way.' The occasional stimulus of a direct request is the kind of challenge many pupils enjoy, and they respond enthusiastically. 'Can you and your partner bat the small ball up and down between you, six times?'

Motivational teaching. Children say that the things that motivate them to take part in physical activities are fun and skill development. They want to enjoy, learn and succeed. The more philosophical among them might also add that feelings of happiness are associated with having something to look forward to; to enjoy; and then to remember with pleasure (and often with pride). This anticipation, realisation and retrospect-inspiring potential of excellent physical education lessons and activities, makes it the favourite subject for many primary school pupils.

Safe Practice and Accident Prevention

In physical education lessons, where a main aim is to contribute to normal, healthy growth and physical development, we must do everything possible to avoid accidents.

Good supervision by the teacher is key to safe practice. He or she must be there with the class at all times, and teaching from positions from which the majority of the class can be seen. This usually means circulating on the outside looking in, with no-one behind his or her back. Good teaching develops skilful, well-controlled, safe movement with pupils wanting to avoid others to ensure that they have space to practise and perform well and not be impeded in any way. The outward expression of this caring attitude we are trying to create is the sensible, unselfish sharing of hall floor space, apparatus and playground, and self-control in avoiding others.

Badly behaved classes who do not respond immediately, or start or stop as requested; who rush around selfishly and noisily disturbing others; who are never quiet in their tongues or body movements; and who do not try to move well, are destructive of any prospects for high standards or lesson enjoyment by the majority and the teacher. A safe environment requires a well-behaved, quiet, attentive and responsive class. Good behaviour must be continually pursued until it becomes the normal, expected way to work in every lesson. There is nothing to talk about, apart from those occasions when comments are requested after a demonstration, or when partners are quietly discussing their response to a challenge.

The hall should be at a good working temperature with windows and doors opened or closed to cope with changing seasons and central heating variations. Potentially dangerous chairs, tables, trolleys, piano or television should be removed or pushed against a wall or into a corner. Floor sockets for receiving securing pins for ropes and climbing frames should be regularly cleared of cleaning substances which harden and block the small sockets.

In playground games lessons, pupils must be trained to remain inside the lines of the grids or netball courts and to avoid running, chasing or dodging into fences, walls, sheds, seats, hutted classrooms, or steps into buildings. In any 'tag' games, pupils must be told 'Touch the person you have caught very gently, never pushing them or causing them to fall or stumble.'

Before the lesson, the teacher checks for sensible, safe clothing with no watches, rings or jewellery whose impact against another child can cause serious scarring or injury; no long trousers that catch heels; no long sleeves that catch thumbs, impeding safe gripping; and no long, un-bunched hair that impedes vision. Indoors, barefoot work is recommended because it is quiet, provides a safe, strong grip on apparatus, enhances the appearance of the work, and enables the little-used muscles of feet and ankles to develop as they grip, balance, support, propel and receive the body weight.

In teaching gymnastic activities, the following safety considerations are important:

❍ In floor and apparatus work, pupils need to be taught the correct, safe, 'squashy' landing after a jump so that they land safely on the balls of the feet, with ankles, knees and hips 'giving' without jarring.

❍ When inverted, with all the weight on their hands, pupils need to be taught to keep fingers pointing forward, arms straight and strong, and head looking forward, not back under arms. Looking back under the arms makes everything appear to be upside down.

❍ On climbing frames, pupils must be told 'Fingers grip over the bar, thumbs grip under the bar, always, for a safe, strong grip.'

Headings When Considering Standards in Physical Education

Physical Education lessons are so visual that most of the following headings can be considered by an interested observer.

○ **Vigorous physical activity**, involving all pupils for most of the lesson, is the most important feature of an excellent lesson.

○ **Responsive pupils, behaving well and obviously enjoying lessons**; working hard to learn and improve skills; and exuding enthusiasm and concentration, are an uplifting feature of high standards.

○ **Enthusiastic teaching, using praise and encouragement warmly**, stimulates pupils to even greater levels of endeavour. Praise is specific, referring to what is pleasing, to inform the pupil being praised and to let others hear and learn. 'Well done, Charlotte. Your balances are still, firm and beautifully stretched.'

○ **Skills, appropriate to the age group**, are taught and developed. There is an impression of skilful, quiet, confident, well-controlled, successful performing with economy of effort. Pupils show understanding by their ability to remember and repeat their movements.

○ **Pupils' behaviour towards one another is excellent**. Undressing and dressing quickly to extend lesson time; safe, unselfish sharing of space and apparatus; working quietly to avoid lessons being stopped because of noise; observing demonstrations with interest and then making helpful, friendly comments; and co-operating well as partners and members of groups and teams, all indicate desirable standards of behaviour.

○ **Varied teaching styles include**:

  a indirect or shared choice teaching

  b direct teaching

  c good and varied use of demonstrations, observations, comments.

○ **Satisfactory time allocation** provides regular, weekly lessons in dance, games and gymnastic activities – a broad programme which also includes athletic activities and swimming for Juniors.

○ **Lesson plans** are in evidence, as a reminder of all parts of the current lesson, and as a reminder of what has been taught, so that the work can be progressed, month by month, throughout the year.

○ **Sensibly dressed pupils** wear shorts, a T shirt or blouse, and plimsolls. Indoors, barefoot work is recommended. As an example, the teacher should at least change into appropriate footwear.

○ **Continuity and progression from year to year** are evident in the way that older pupils work harder for longer at increasingly difficult activities, demonstrating skill and versatility.

○ **An awareness of safe practice and accident prevention** is evident in the way that pupils share the limited space. The correct way to lift, carry and use apparatus, land, move, roll, support and use the body generally, are regularly mentioned.

A Suggested Way to Start a First Lesson with a New Class

Unless taught otherwise, pupils travel round the hall or the playground in an anti-clockwise circle, all following the person in front of them. If one pupil slows down or stops suddenly, the next can bump into that person, possibly knocking him or her over, causing an angry upset and a disturbance.

By travelling and confining themselves within this circle, a class fails to use all the possible room or playground space, depriving themselves of enough space to travel freely in different directions, and to join several actions together, on the spot or travelling about. Also, with everyone travelling round in a circle, sometimes side by side, pairs of less well-behaved pupils can be so close together that their poor behaviour, expressed in talking, not listening, slow responses, and noisy, poor performances, completely upsets the teacher's aim to give the class an enjoyable, lively, quiet, thoughtful and co-operative start to the lesson and the year's programme.

By continually making the whole class listen for the signal 'Stop!', we force them to pay attention, listen, and respond quickly.

Suggested pre-start to the lesson

1 Please show me your very best walking...go! Visit every part of the room, the sides, the ends, corners, as well as the middle. Swing your arms strongly and step out smartly.

2 When I call 'Stop!', show me how quickly you can stop and stand perfectly still. Keep walking smartly and visiting all parts of the room. Stop! Stand still!

3 If you are standing too near a piece of apparatus, like James by the piano, or too near someone else, like Leroy and Emily, please take one step into a big space all by yourself. Go!

4 When you start walking this time, travel along straight lines, never following anyone. If you find yourself behind someone, change direction and continue along a new straight line, following no-one. Ready? Go!

5 Come on. March briskly and smartly and pretend you are leaving footprints in every part of the room. When I call 'Stop!' you will stop immediately and then take a step into your own space if you are near apparatus or another person. Stop!

6 In our next practice, listen for my 'Stop!' and show me that no-one is standing behind another person, looking towards that person's back, following them. Go!

7 Stop! Stand still, after moving onto your own space if necessary. Now show your very best running, with the emphasis on lifting your heels, knees and hands to keep your running soft, silent and strong – and, of course, travelling along straight lines, never following anyone.

8 Stop! Be still! This half of the class stand with feet apart, arms folded, to watch this other half doing their very best running. Look out for and tell me later about anyone whose running you liked and be able to tell me what you liked about it. The running half...ready...go! Do not pick anyone who is following someone, or anyone who is not lifting heels, knees or arms strongly. Please watch carefully.

9 Stop! Watchers, whose running did you like. Yes, Liam?

10   I (Liam) liked Nathalie's running because she used her eyes well, looking for spaces, and she seemed to float along beautifully and easily, with heels, knees and hands being lifted high.

11 Thank you very much, Liam, for that excellent answer. Now let's look at Nathalie to see and learn from the good things mentioned by Liam. Please run again, Nathalie.

12 (Repeat with the other half working and the other half observing and commenting.)

Potential Cross-Curricular Outcomes of Physical Education Lessons for Infants

Language Many teachers recognise the valuable contribution that physical education lessons can make to language development and a clearer understanding of the meanings of words. Hearing, reading and writing are the usual relationships between pupils and words. In physical education lessons, pupils do, experience and feel the actions words concerned. Clear demonstrations by the teacher or a pupil also lead to a greater understanding of the exact meanings of action words.

In Reception, Games Lesson 1, for example, there are: visit, follow, run, jump, balance, throw, catch, aim, pick, swing, show, place, land, balance, slide, practise, send, fly, roll, head, bounce, bat. Jog, dodge, mark, dribble, touch, bowl, receive, chase, sprint and skip are also frequently used in games lessons.

In a typical gymnastic activities lesson, pupils will also experience, understand and feel the meanings of the many prepositions used, for example, in Year 1, Lesson 5: around, up to, under, across, along, near, on, above. Beside, beneath, towards, over, through, astride, off, away, are also frequently used in gymnastics lessons.

Adverbs describe the quality or degree of effort in an action as in Year 2, Dance Lesson 2: slowly, well, smartly, carefully, beautifully, springy, lively, firmly, particularly. Quickly, gently, strongly, smoothly, stiffly, loosely, loudly, quietly, explosively, vigorously, are also used frequently in dance lessons.

Writing/discussion Still within language, pupils can be challenged to recall 'The part(s) of the gymnastics lesson where I felt (choose one of), for example, excited, pleased, surprised, tired, proud, anxious, hot, breathless, strong, stretched, unsure, was/were...' They can be asked to explain why they were experiencing the feelings they listed.

A mountaineer once said 'When I climb, I can feel life effervescing within me.' A pupil who has just completed a rope climb for the first time; or done a beautifully stretched, controlled cartwheel; or completed their own created dance or gymnastics sequence with complete control from start to finish; or outwitted a games opponent before going on to score, will be experiencing intense excitement, pride and pleasure, deserving of the opportunity to try to produce an eloquent expression about what might have been an unforgettable event.

Art Pupils can be asked 'Can you draw the gymnastic action or actions that gave you the most pleasure or excitement in today's lesson? Under your drawing, can you write in a few words why you were pleased or excited?'

Physical education can also contribute to pupils':

○ **spiritual development** through helping them gain a sense of achievement and develop positive attitudes towards themselves

○ **moral development** through helping pupils gain a sense of fair play based on rules and the conventions of activities; and develop positive sporting behaviour, knowing how to conduct themselves in sporting competition

○ **social development** through helping pupils develop social skills in activities involving co-operation and collaboration, responsibility, personal commitment, loyalty and teamwork, and considering the social importance of physical activity, sport and dance.

Gymnastic Activities

Introduction to Gymnastic Activities

Gymnastic Activities is the indoor lesson that includes varied floorwork on a clear floor, unimpeded by apparatus, followed by varied apparatus work which should take up just over half of the lesson time. Ideally, the portable apparatus will have been positioned around the sides and ends of the room, near to where it will be used, before lessons start in the morning or afternoon. This allows each of the seven or eight mixed infant groups, or the five or six mixed junior groups of pupils to lift, carry and position their apparatus in a very short time, because no set will need to be moved more than 3–5 metres. The lesson is traditionally of 30 minutes duration.

  The following pages aim, first of all, to produce a sense of staff-room unity regarding the nature of good practice and high standards in teaching Gymnastic Activities lessons. Without this sense of unity among the teachers concerned, there is no continuity of aims, expectations or programme, and there will be a less than satisfactory level of achievement. Secondly, the following pages provide a full scheme of work for Gymnastic Activities. There is a lesson plan and accompanying pages of detailed explanatory notes for every month, designed to help teachers and schools with ideas for lessons that are progressive.

Why We Teach Gymnastic Activities

Ideally, the expressions of intent known as 'Aims' should represent the combined views of all the staff.

Aim 1 To inspire vigorous physical activity to promote normal healthy growth and physical development. Physical Education is most valuable when pupils' participation is enthusiastic, vigorous and wholehearted. All subsequent aims for a good programme depend on achieving this first aim.

Aim 2 To teach physical skills to develop skilful, well-controlled, versatile movement. We want pupils to enjoy moving well, safely and confidently. Physical Education makes a unique contribution to a child's physical development because the activities are experienced at first hand by doing them.

Aim 3 To help pupils become good learners as well as good movers. Knowledge, understanding and learning are achieved through a combination of doing, feeling and experiencing physical activity. Pupils are challenged to think for themselves, making decisions about their actions.

Aim 4 To develop pupils' self-confidence and self-esteem by appreciating the importance of physical achievement; by helping them to achieve; and by recognising and sharing such achievement with others.

Aim 5 To develop desirable social qualities, helping pupils get on well with one another by bringing them together in mutual endeavours. Friendly, co-operative, close relationships are an ever-present feature of Physical Education lessons.

Aim 6 To provide opportunities for exciting, almost adventurous actions (particularly climbing, swinging, balancing, jumping and landing) and vigorous exercise – seldom experienced away from school. We want our pupils to use these lessons as outlets for their energy and we want them to believe that exercise is good for you and your heart, and makes you feel and look better. We aim to encourage participation in a healthy lifestyle, long after pupils have left school.

The Gymnastic Activities Lesson Plan for Infants – 30 minutes

One answer to the question 'What do we teach in a gymnastic activities lesson?' might be – 'All the natural activities and ways of moving of which the body is capable and which, if practised safely and wholeheartedly, ensure normal healthy growth and physical development.'

It has been said that 'What you don't use, you lose.' Most pupils hardly ever strenuously use their natural capacity for vigorous running, jumping and landing from a height; rolling in different directions; balancing on a variety of body parts; upending to take their weight on their hands; gripping, climbing and swinging on a rope; hanging, swinging or circling on a bar; or whole body bending, stretching, arching and twisting. These natural movements and actions should be present in every gymnastic activities lesson, ensuring that pupils do not lose the ability to do them and that their physical development does not diminish.

A teacher's determination to inspire the class to use and not lose their natural physicality can be strengthened by observing how many children are collected in cars at the school gates. They are then transported home to their after school, house-bound, sedentary home lives.

Floorwork (12 minutes) starts the lesson and includes:

○ Activities for the legs, exploring and developing the many actions possible when travelling on feet, and ways to jump and land.

○ Activities for the body, including the many ways to bend, stretch, rock, roll, twist, curl, turn, and the ways in which body parts receive, support and transfer the body weight in travelling and balancing.

○ Activities for the arms and shoulders, the least used parts of our body. We strengthen them by using them to hold all or part of the body weight on the spot or moving. This strength is needed in gripping, climbing, hanging, swinging and circling, and in levering on to and across apparatus, supported by the hands alone.

Apparatus Work (16 minutes) is the climax of the lesson, making varied, unique and challenging demands on pupils whose whole body – legs, arms and shoulders, back and abdominal muscles – must work hard because of the more difficult tasks:

○ travelling on hands and feet, over, under, across and around obstacles, as well as vertically, often supported only on hands

○ jumping and landing from greater heights

○ rolling on to, along, from and across apparatus

○ balancing on high or narrow surfaces

○ upending to take all body weight on hands on apparatus above floor level

○ gripping, swinging, climbing and circling on ropes and bars.

Final Floor Activity (2 minutes) after the apparatus has been returned to its starting places around the sides, ends and corners of the hall, brings the whole class together again in a simple activity based on the lesson's main emphasis or theme. After the bustle of apparatus removal – the swishing of ropes along trackways, the creaking of climbing frames being wheeled away, the bumping of benches, planks, boxes and trestles – there is a quiet, calm, thoughtful and focused ending.

Three Ways to Teach Apparatus Work

1 **(Easiest Method) Pupils use all the apparatus freely, as they respond to tasks that relate to the lesson theme**. Several challenges provide non-stop apparatus work for infants and juniors. Pupils are stationary only when watching a demonstration, having a teaching point emphasised, or when being given the next task. This method is normally used with infant classes, because they are able to visit and use all pieces of apparatus, including their favourites – ropes and climbing frames.

   'Show me a still balance and beautifully stretched body shape on each piece of apparatus.' (Body shape awareness and balance)

   'Show me how you can approach each piece of apparatus going forward and leave going sideways.' (Space awareness – directions)

   'Leader, show your partner one touch only on each piece of apparatus, then off to the next piece.' (Partner work)

2 **Groups stay and work at one set of apparatus**. Repetition helps pupils improve and remember a series of linked actions. The task is the same for all groups, based on the lesson theme.

   'Make your hands important in arriving on, and your feet important in leaving the apparatus.' (Body parts awareness)

   'Can you include swings on to and off apparatus; a swing into a roll; and a swing to take all the weight on your hands?' (Swinging)

   'Travel from opposite sides, up to, on, along and from the apparatus, to finish in your partner's starting place.' (Partner work)

   Groups rotate to the next apparatus after about five minutes and will work at three sets in a lesson, rotating clockwise one lesson, and anti-clockwise the next, to meet all apparatus every two lessons.

3 **Each group practises a different, specific skill on each piece of apparatus – balancing, rolling, climbing, for example**. This method of teaching is more difficult than the other two because it needs more technical knowledge, and because the teacher is giving five or six sets of instructions instead of one. As it is a direct challenge to 'skills hungry' pupils, it is very popular.

   Benches 'At upturned benches, slowly balance and walk forward. Look straight ahead. Feel for the bench before you step on it.'

   Ropes 'Grip strongly with hands together and feet crossed. Can you take one hand off, while swinging, to prove a good foot grip?'

   Low cross box 'A face vault is like a high bunny jump to cross the box, as you twist over, facing the box top all the way.'

   Climbing frames 'Travel by moving hands only, then feet only.'

   Mats 'Roll sideways with body curled small and then with body long and stretched' (log roll).

   Groups rotate to the next piece of apparatus after about five minutes, rotating clockwise one lesson, and anti-clockwise the next lesson, meeting all apparatus every two lessons.

Organising Groups for Infant School Apparatus Work

The recommended system for ensuring that apparatus can be lifted, carried and placed in position, quickly and easily, needs the co-operation of all the teachers. Before lessons start in the morning or afternoon, the portable apparatus is placed around the sides and ends of the hall near to where it will be used. Each group of pupils will thus only have to carry it 2–3 metres. A well-trained class can have the apparatus in place in 30 seconds. After all lessons are finished each day, as much of the apparatus as possible should remain in the hall, in corners, against or on the platform, or at the sides and ends of the room. Mats can be stored vertically behind climbing frames, benches and boxes.

Groups of four pupils are appropriate for infant school apparatus work and the organisation into the seven or eight groups is done in the first lesson in September. Pupils are told 'These are your groups and starting places for apparatus work.' For the four or five lessons, the same groups go to the same starting places, becoming expert in lifting, carrying and placing their apparatus. At the start of the school year, groups are taught how to lift, carry and place the various pieces of apparatus. For example, at a bench, box or nesting table group, 'Stand, one at each end and one at each side. Bend your knees, put your hands under your side of the apparatus with arms straight. Stand up and lift carefully. Carry it to here, please, then bend your knees to put it down quietly.' The teacher shows them a position, a few metres away from where they started. 'Liam and Nathalie, please bring your mat now, and put it beside the bench.'

At the end of the lesson, the class is asked to go and stand beside the apparatus they brought out. After the apparatus has been returned to its starting places at the sides or ends of the room, groups should be praised for the 'quiet, safe and sensible way you all moved your apparatus' and reminded 'Please remember your own starting place for apparatus next week.'

Positioning of Apparatus During Lessons

The teacher needs to provide varied actions and physical demands as pupils progress from apparatus to apparatus, meeting a challenging, interesting series of settings. The typical spread of eight or nine simple sets of apparatus might include:

- bench and mat
- trestle, inclined plank and mat
- ropes frame
- nesting table and mat
- bottom section of box and mat

- bench and mat
- two trestles, plank to link trestles and mat
- climbing frames
- top section of two-section box and mat
- pyramid boxes, linking plank and mats

A safe environment is ensured by providing:

- mats where pupils are expected to land from a height
- mats that are well away from walls, windows, doors or other obstacles such as a piano, trolley chairs, and well away from the landing areas of adjacent apparatus
- height and width of apparatus that are appropriate for the age of the class – not too narrow to balance on, and not too high to jump from.

Mats are used to cushion a landing from a height and to roll on. We do not use mats under ropes or around climbing frames because we do not ask pupils to jump down from a height. If mats are placed around climbing frames, pupils often behave in a foolhardy way, enticed into dangerous jumping.

Fixed and portable apparatus

Apparatus referred to in the lesson plans that follow, and shown in the examples of simple and larger apparatus groupings, include the following items:

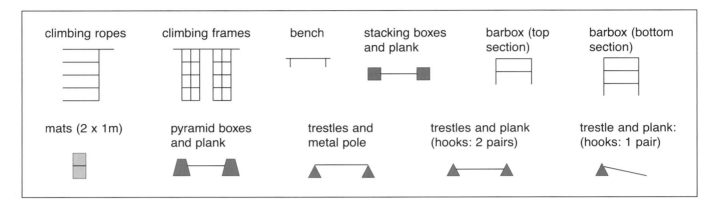

Minimum number recommended:

○ 12 mats 2 × 1 m

○ 3 benches

○ 1 barbox that can be divided into two smaller boxes by lifting off the top section. The lower section should have a platform top

○ 1 pair stacking boxes, 48 × 48 cm base, 33 cm high; and one 2.4 m plank

○ 1 pair pyramid boxes, 78 cm high, 60 cm long, 53 cm wide at base tapering to 38 cm wide at top, and one 2.4 m plank

○ 1 pair of 1 m, 1.06 m, 1.4 m trestles

○ 2 planks with two pairs of hooks

○ 2 planks with one pair of hooks

○ 1 3 m metal pole

simple layout 1

simple layout 2

larger groups layout

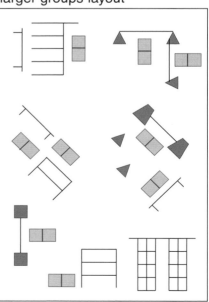

A Pattern for Teaching and Improving a Gymnastic Activities Action

Using 'Travelling' as an example

1 **Quickly into action**. With few words, clearly explain the task and challenge the class to start. For example 'Can you plan to travel, using your feet, sometimes going forwards, and sometimes in another direction?'

2 **While class is working**. Emphasise the main points, one at a time. There is no need to stop a well-behaved class who are working quietly every time you need to make a teaching point. 'Find quiet spaces in all parts of the room – the sides, ends, corners, as well as the middle.' 'Work so quietly that I can't hear you.' 'Travel on straight lines, never curving round, following someone.' 'Look over your shoulder if going backwards.'

3 **Identify and praise good work while class is working**. The teacher needs to circulate round the outside of the room, looking in to see as much of the work as possible. 'Well done, John. I liked your skipping forwards and bouncing sideways.' 'Emily, your hopscotch is a great idea.' 'Sarah, your slow, careful running backwards with high knees lifting, is a neat, safe way to travel.'

4 **Demonstrations accompanied by teacher comment are the quickest way to increase the class repertoire**. It saves time if the demonstrators have been told what aspect of movement they are about to be asked to demonstrate. 'We will be looking at your beautifully stretched body in your jumps, and the soft, quiet way you let your knees and ankles give when you land.' 'Stop and watch Michael's lively, quiet bouncing with feet parting and closing, going sideways. And look at Sophie's galloping backwards with a strong arm swing.'
   Beware of stopping the class too often to use a demonstration. Make these stoppages brief, between 12 and 15 seconds.

5 **Further practice should follow a demonstration with reminders of the good things seen**. Pupils enjoy copying something they never thought of trying – particularly when it has been warmly praised and approved of. 'Thank you for those excellent demonstrations. Practise again, and try to improve your travelling by using something of what you have just seen. Use your whole body strongly, but quietly. Your feet can travel together or apart, or one after the other.'

6 **Demonstrations (by an individual, a small group or half of the class) with follow-up comments by the pupils are used to let pupils reflect on and evaluate their own and others' performances**. Such comments and judgements guide the next stage of planning for improvement. 'Watch this group of four working and tell me which travelling actions you like best, and say which directions you saw being used.' This is followed by a brief look at the pupils mentioned.

7 **Demonstrators and those making comments are thanked and more class practice lets them try some of the good things seen**. Beware of using demonstrations with follow-up comments more than once or twice in the lesson because they are time-consuming.

Progressing Gymnastic Activities over the 4 or 5 weeks of the Lesson's Development

Using 'Stepping' as an example of an activity to be developed

Lessons 1 and 2

a Concentrate on the **'What?'**, the actions, their correct form, and how the body parts concerned are working.

'Can you step quietly and neatly, visiting all parts of the room? Travel on straight lines, never following anyone.'

'Which parts of the foot can support you? Tip toes, insides or outsides? Long or short steps or a mixture?'

'Can you vary the idea of stepping, not always passing your feet?' (Chasse, crossover, toes down and swing.)

b Insist on good, clear body shapes to make everything look better and be more demanding.

'Step out nice and tall as you travel. Can you show me your clear arms, legs and body shape? Are you long and stretched or is there a body shape change somewhere?'

Lessons 2 and 3

Concentrate on the **'Where?'** of the movement, adding variety and quality by good use of own and whole floor space, directions and levels.

'Can you sometimes step on the spot, (particularly when you are in a crowded area) and sometimes use the whole room space – sides, corners, ends as well as middle.'

'Stepping actions sideways and backwards can be interesting – sliding, stepping-closing (chasse) or cross-stepping over, as well as feet passing normally. The leading leg can swing in many directions.'

Lessons 3 and 4

Consider the **'How?'** of the movements and the way that changes of speed and effort (force) might make the work look more controlled and neat, as well as giving them greater variety, contrast and interest.

'Within your stepping, can you include a change of speed? It might be slow, slow; quick, quick, 3, 4; slow, slow. Flat, flat; tip toes, tip toes, 3, 4; flat, flat.. This is interesting if a change of direction accompanies the speed change. Side, slow, slow; forward, quick, quick, 3, 4; side, slow, slow.' 'Can you make parts of your travelling small, soft, quiet, and make parts bigger, firmer, stronger?' (On the spot, keep it soft, 1, 2, 3, 4; on the move, big strong strides, 1, 2, 3, 4.)

Lessons 4 or Lessons 4 and 5

Ask for **sequences** that draw together all the practising, learning, adapting and remembering that have taken place during the previous lessons and aim for almost non-stop action, working harder for longer with enthusiasm, understanding and concentration.

'In your 3 or 4 part sequence, can you include: varied stepping actions, interesting use of space, and a change of speed or force somewhere?'

The Use of Themes in Teaching Gymnastic Activities

Week after week, month after month, the teacher and class come into the school hall and see the same apparatus, apparently offering the same limited set of activities every time. In dance, we continually move on to learning and performing new dances and building a huge repertoire. In games, the new seasons bring their different sports and the varied games implements provide an interesting and exciting range – including new games created by the teacher and pupils.

Gymnastic activities lessons are made different through applying a new idea, emphasis or theme each month. We do not simply 'do' the basic action. We do it, focusing on a particular aspect of movement, to improve in understanding and versatility, as well as in competence. A theme is a particular aspect of movement chosen by the teacher as a focal point around which to build a series of lessons.

At the very beginning of the series of four or five lessons during which an individual lesson is repeated, it is recommended that the pupils are 'put in the picture' regarding their lesson's main aims or emphases. In cases where they are going to be assessed on the outcome of the lesson, it is essential to explain to them what new skills, knowledge and understanding they will be expected to demonstrate. Identifying the lesson theme or main emphasis to the class is also a way for the teacher to put him or herself 'in the picture' about the main objectives of the lesson and to focus on them.

Start of year themes with a new class will have an emphasis on good behaviour; sensible, safe sharing of floor and apparatus space; immediate responses to commands and challenges set by the teacher; establishing a tradition of wholehearted, vigorous effort and a co-operative attitude towards one's classmates; and co-operating with others to lift, carry and place apparatus quietly, sensibly and safely.

A suggested set of six progressive themes for a month to month programme

1   **Body parts awareness** for better controlled, safer, more correct activity. 'Show me varied ways to travel, using one foot, both feet, or one foot after the other.'

2   **Body shape awareness** for improved poise, better posture and firmer body tension. 'Can you run and jump up high with feet together and long, straight legs?'

3   **Space awareness** for improved variety, quality and interest, and safer practising. 'Can you travel all round the room, using feet only, sometimes going forwards, and sometimes sideways?'

4   **Effort awareness** for more interesting contrasts, better quality and stronger work. 'As you travel in a variety of ways can you include actions that are small, light and gentle, and actions that are large, lively and strong?'

5   **Sequences** for longer, harder, versatile work, stamping it with own personality. 'Make up a sequence you can remember, of three or four joined-up actions and changing body shapes on different body parts.' (Standing, kneeling, lying, sitting, upended on shoulders, arched on back or front.)

6   **Partner work** for new, enjoyable, sociable, more demanding experiences not possible on one's own, and to extend movement understanding because you need to recognise partner's actions. 'Stand, facing each other. Can you, with a little bend of knees as a start signal, bounce at the same speed? Can you do opposites, with one going up as the other comes down?'

A Progressive Series of Themes for a Gymnastic Activities Programme

An example from parts of lessons based on 'ways to travel'

Floorwork

Apparatus Work

Theme 1. Body parts awareness – for neater, better controlled, safer, more correct activity.

a Show me varied ways to travel, using one foot, both feet, or one foot after the other. As you travel about, slowly, using hands and feet, can you make different parts of your body go first?

a Plan to visit many pieces of apparatus. 'Feel' the different ways your hands and feet can:
  1 support you (for example, as you hang, swing, crawl, circle, roll, slide, skip, jump, balance.)
  2 go from apparatus to apparatus, putting hands on the apparatus, and show me a bunny jump with straight arms and well bent legs.

Theme 2. Body shape awareness – for improved poise, better posture and firmer body tension.

a Can you run and jump up high with feet together and long, straight legs?
b Can you run and jump up high to show me a wide shape like a star?

a Run quietly round the room, not touching any apparatus. When I call 'Stop!', show me a clear body shape on the nearest apparatus.
b Run round again and when I stop you next time, show me a different, firm body shape.

Theme 3. Space awareness – for improved variety, quality and interest, and safer practising.

a Can you travel all round the room, using feet only, sometimes forwards, and sometimes going sideways? Which are best for going forwards? Which are best for going sideways?

a Can you arrive on and leave the apparatus at different places and in different ways?
b Take weight on hands, with straight arms and bent legs. Bring feet down slowly in a new floor space.

Theme 4. Effort awareness – for more interesting contrasts, better quality, and stronger work.

As you travel in a variety of ways, can you include actions that are small, light and gentle, and actions that are large, lively and strong?

Travel freely. Show me strong, firm balances on apparatus that contrast with easier travelling actions in between. Can you do a vigorous upward jump, off, then a soft 'giving' landing.

Theme 5. Sequences – for longer, harder, versatile work, stamping it with own personality.

Work in a small floor space and show me two or more ways to travel on feet or feet and hands. Can you give each action a name? Show me a still start and finish.

Start in a still, nicely balanced position on the floor. Travel on to a piece of apparatus and show me a neat, still balance position.

Theme 6. Partner work – for new, more exciting experiences not possible on your own.

Follow your leader's varied travelling.

Follow on to and along each piece of apparatus.

National Curriculum Requirements for Gymnastics Activities – Key Stage 1: The Main Features

'The government believes that two hours of physical activity a week, including the National Curriculum for Physical Education and extra-curricular activities, should be an aspiration for all schools. This applies to all stages.'

Programme of study
Pupils should be taught to:

a perform basic skills in travelling; being still; finding and using space both on the floor and using apparatus

b develop the range of their skills and actions (for example, balancing, jumping and landing, climbing, rolling)

c link skills and actions in short movement phrases

d create and perform short, linked sequences that show a clear beginning, middle and end with contrasts in direction, level and speed.

Attainment target
Pupils should be able to demonstrate that they can:

a select and use skills, actions and ideas appropriately, applying them with control and co-ordination

b copy, explore and remember skills, and link them in ways that suit the activities

c observe and talk about differences between their own and others' performances and use this understanding to improve their own performance.

Main NC headings when considering assessment of progression and expectation

Planning thoughtfully precedes the performance. Pupils think ahead to what their response will be, trying to 'see' the intended outcome. Evidence of satisfactory planning is seen in:

a sensible, safe judgements

b an obvious understanding of what was asked for

c good use of the movement elements that enhance and provide quality, variety and contrast.

Performing and improving performance is the main aim and evident as pupils:

a work hard, concentrating on the main features of the task

b practise to show safe, skilful, controlled activity

c demonstrate that they can remember and repeat the actions.

Linking actions together, with control, into 'sentences of movement' with a still start and finish and a flowing middle, provides a basis for progression, and is evident as pupils:

a work harder for longer

b work more confidently

c show greater use of the space, shape and effort elements that provide attractive variety and contrast in sequences.

Reflecting and making judgements is evident as pupils:

a describe the most important features of a demonstration

b suggest ways to improve

c self-evaluate and act upon their own reflections.

Year 2 Gymnastic Activities Programme

Pupils should be able to:

Autumn	Spring	Summer
1 Respond quickly to instructions, performing whole-heartedly, vigorously and safely.	1 Show ability and desire to respond safely and quickly to tasks in varied ways.	1 Respond to set tasks with confidence and enthusiasm.
2 Work, almost non-stop, trying to do neat, quiet performances.	2 Practise whole-heartedly and continuously, focusing on actions, body parts used and good spacing.	2 Manage the body in a well-controlled way, using the full range of movement in the joints and muscles concerned.
3 Share floor and apparatus space unselfishly with others.	3 Balance well on varied parts and show good, firm shapes.	3 Show good space awareness – knowing how to slow down, speed up, pause to accommodate and not impede others sharing the space.
4 Pursue competence, originality and versatility by thoughtful, well-planned practising.	4 Be effort and speed aware, feeling good body tension for a controlled performance.	4 Use varied speeds and effort for more spectacular performances – explosive jumps, gentle rolls, firm balances, slow stretches and curls, strong climbs.
5 In travelling and flight, use vigorous, varied take-off and landing actions, using arms well for balance.	5 Be body-shape aware in stillness, balance and travelling.	5 Co-operate with a partner, travelling together, copying each other, observing and commenting, and working in unison.
6 Support body weight on hands safely with straight arms, head forwards, and just the right amount of effort in the push.	6 Be keen to improve, working hard, alone, and with partner.	6 Show a well-practised expertise in lifting, carrying, placing apparatus, quickly, quietly and safely with others.
7 Include firm, still balances within sequences as contrast to continuous, vigorous action.	7 Co-operate with a partner to mirror, contrast, lead, follow.	7 Feel that they have progressed and understand the nature of the progress, e.g. excellent jumps and landings; varied rolls; weight on hands with confidence; smooth rolls; and well-linked sentences.
8 Be body-shape aware to progress the work and improve its style.	8 Work, almost non-stop, with no queuing or impeding others.	8 Approach, mount, travel on and dismount from apparatus, responding to set tasks with confidence and enthusiasm.
9 Be body-parts aware, 'feeling' how the parts are working.	9 Work hard to deserve praise and stamp work with own special style and personality.	9 Observe demonstrations and comment on actions and any features worth copying or learning from.
10 Demonstrate increasing control and understanding by including direction and level changes.	10 Plan and perform sequences of actions linked neatly, quietly, with control and poise.	10 Recognise the effects of physical activity on bodies – deep breathing, faster pulse rate, feeling hot, becoming exhausted.
11 Be reminded of the correct, safe way to lift, carry and place apparatus, working with others.	11 Show ability to approach, mount, travel on and leave apparatus without impeding others, and with interesting, versatile contrasts such as jumps, rolls, balances and inversion.	
12 Link movements with control.	12 Observe performances with interest and suggest ways in which they might be improved.	
13 Observe a performance and comment on what was well done and worth copying.		

Lesson Plan 1 • 30 minutes
September

Emphasis on: *(a) unselfish co-operation in sharing floor and apparatus space; (b) immediate responses to instructions; (c) variety in travelling on floor and apparatus, using feet, feet and hands, and other body surfaces.*

Floorwork
12 minutes

Legs

1 Can you walk, run, jump and land without stopping, and carry on with your walking again?

2 Because you are travelling non-stop, look ahead and plan to walk, then run just the right distance to let you do your lively jump in a good space.

3 Can you show me other ways to travel, using legs only? (For example, skip, bounce, gallop, hopscotch, slip sideways.)

Body

1 Lie down on your back, front or side. Stretch your body out fully, reaching your arms above your head and pointing your toes. Can you travel by changing to a curled shape? Try it again. (For example, to lying curled on one side after sideways roll.)

2 From your bent shape, can you now travel to a new supporting part, with your body stretched again? (For example, roll on to knees, stretch arms forwards and up above head.)

3 Now can you do one more curl and stretch for me? (For example, roll to a sitting, curled position, then rock back to stretched shoulder balance.) Go back to your starting position and try again.

Arms

1 Look for a clear space each time, then travel slowly on hands and feet. Try to show me your actions clearly.

2 Are you sometimes using hands and feet apart, and sometimes closer together? Which way is easier?

3 Can you travel by moving hands only and then feet only, stretching, then curling your body?

Apparatus Work
16 minutes

1 Using feet only, travel to all parts of the room where you see good spaces, but do not touch any apparatus.

2 Can you do your floorwork, walking, running and jumping without stopping? (For example, walking across, under, through, in and out of apparatus; running on floor, across mats, astride benches; jumping over mats, benches, low planks.)

3 Use your feet only to bring you on to, take you along, then bring you off the apparatus. Plan to show me a good variety of actions. (For example, step, jump or bounce on; walk, skip, high jump from.)

4 Now you may use both hands and feet to take you travelling up to, on, along and from the apparatus. Travel slowly enough for me to see your different actions clearly.

5 Earlier, in our floorwork, we travelled by going from a stretch to a curl. Can you now travel on floor and all apparatus, changing from a long, stretched body to one that is curled up small? (For example, up and down the climbing frames; on two ropes with a stretched swing to a curled landing; under and on poles, planks, benches and boxes; rolling across mats.)

Final Floor Activity
2 minutes

Show me one way to travel, using your feet silently.

Teaching notes and NC guidance
Development over 4 lessons

Floorwork

Legs

1. Pupils will jump, land and be still, if it is not emphasised that we 'land and keep going!'

2. The jump is the main feature, and some pupils will need to be dissuaded from running long distances without a jump.

3. Much teacher commentary on activities observed and selected demonstrations will inspire the variety aimed for in this lesson.

Body

1. It helps to produce a quick response if the teacher suggests a starting, stretched position from which it is easy to curl up.

2. If the class are slow to respond, once again the teacher can suggest a next move which satisfies the set task.

3. From needing an assisted start to the sequence, the class, week by week, will begin to introduce their own ideas for supporting parts, and even include different levels.

Arms

1. Insist on 'slow travelling, using both hands and feet. No quick scampering!' Rushing around in and out of one another is common, but puts little weight on hands and does little to build skill, strength or understanding.

2. 'Hands and feet apart' can mean a cartwheel, as well as the travel with hands and feet both supporting down near the floor. Wide hands and feet, with a long body near to floor, is difficult to support. Hands and feet close in a high arch is also difficult.

3. You can have front (the usual), back or one side to the floor as you move hands only, then feet only.

Apparatus Work

1. Travel everywhere, except on apparatus. To test pupils' 'immediate responses' and their 'unselfish sharing of floor', the teacher can call 'Stop!' Praise those who respond immediately and those who are in a space, well away from others.

2. With good planning and thinking ahead, pupils can travel non-stop, walking, running and jumping as appropriate.

3. 'Feet only travelling' means that we cannot use ropes, and can only step on and off the climbing frames from a low height. Praise neat, quiet actions with good body shapes and good use of arms for any balancing from jumps.

4. 'Hands and feet travelling now' brings all apparatus into use. Discourage queues at favourite ropes and climbing frames, and encourage a continuous circulation from piece to adjacent piece.

5. Revision of the floorwork, plus new work now possible on floor and apparatus, will challenge pupils' planning ability as they climb, roll, swing, circle, vault, travel, while thinking about their changing body shapes. It will also challenge the teacher to be aware of what is going on and to comment on and demonstrate it, if it seems a good addition to the class repertoire.

Final Floor Activity

The teacher can say 'If I close my eyes and ask you to travel on your feet so silently that I cannot hear you, what action or actions will you choose to use?'

Lesson Plan 2 • 30 minutes
October

Emphasis on: *(a) controlling the body shape to enhance the appearance of a performance and to make you work harder; (b) observing demonstrations with interest, and describing the actions enjoyed and any special features.*

Floorwork
12 minutes

Legs

1   Stand tall and still on tiptoes. Run and jump up into a beautifully stretched jump with straight arms high above head. Land softly and show a still, tall finish.

2   Try one- and two-footed take-offs to see which gives you more height and time to make your big stretch in the air.

3   You can land with feet apart, side to side, or one in front of the other. Or you can land with one foot after the other, which slows you down nicely for your neat, still finish. On landing, feel how straight arms help your balance.

Body

1   Can you keep at least one hand on the floor and show me how to join together different body movements and shapes, such as bending, stretching, twisting and arching?

2   If you are short of ideas, lie on your back with hands on the floor and body wide stretched. Now come up to sitting curled; change to side, falling stretched on one hand and one foot; put the top (non-supporting) hand under the other arm and twist to lie on back again.

3   I will find your linking movements interesting. Show me slowly and clearly how you change from shape to shape.

Arms

1   With one, both or alternate hands on the floor, can you lift your legs in the air, stretching them long and high?

2   Your arms will also be long and straight for a safe, strong support.

Apparatus Work
16 minutes

1   Run silently in and out of one another without touching any apparatus except mats. When I call 'Stop!' show me a clear, still body shape on the nearest apparatus. 'Stop!'

2   When I stop you next time, try to show me a body shape that contrasts with one of the others on the apparatus with you.

3   Travel up to your first piece of apparatus and arrive on it with your body curled up strongly. (For example, hanging from pole, rope or plank; crouched small on feet on climbing frame or box top; curled on shoulders on mat, plank or box; lying on one side on plank, box or mat.) From this still start, change to travelling on your apparatus and try to include clear body shapes as you go. After you leave the apparatus, show me a still, tall, stretched finishing position.

4   Stay at your number one apparatus and show me a sequence that includes: (a) strong leg and arm travelling actions; (b) varied body movements – bending, stretching, curling, twisting; (c) a variety of clear body shapes, both still and moving; (d) a still starting and finishing position on the floor away from the apparatus.

Final Floor Activity
2 minutes

How many travelling actions can you do with a leg or legs nicely stretched?

Teaching notes and NC guidance
Development over 4 lessons

Floorwork

Legs

1   Good posture and tall, erect, unsagging carriage are commented on right from the start of the lesson. A whole-hearted effort is needed to produce this clearly stretched, whole-body shape in flight – and whole-heartedness is always one of our aims.

2   Only a short, 3–4 metre run is needed to prepare you for the settle and upwards spring, which is strongest from both feet.

3   A slow, controlled landing is easier if feet land one after the other, slowing you down gradually. Straight arms forwards or sideways act to balance you.

Body

1   The body movement part of the floorwork is often the most difficult to get started, because the actions and movements are unusual and not often experienced. All the more important, therefore, to encourage these big body movements in order to retain our whole body suppleness and strength.

2   A directed start by the teacher helps the class to understand the task and gives them starting points from which to develop their own ideas during future lessons.

3   All sequences of joined-up movements need linking actions. Skill in linking actions is as admirable and worth praising as good performances of the main movements.

Arms

1   Ensure that all pupils have good space behind them to let them kick up a leg into their cartwheels or handstands. The kicking-up leg is straight and stays stretched during the move.

2   Straight arms tend to stay unbending and strong. Any 'give' in the arm while up-ended can easily cause a collapse.

Apparatus Work

1   Encourage running 'in and out of one another' to and from all directions, rather than all following all in one big circle. The 'Stop!' lets the teacher check on the quality of pupils' spacing and their immediate response to a signal.

2   If there are four or five sharing a set of apparatus, the one you choose to contrast with might in turn be concentrating on another. We hope to see a variety of supporting body parts, not always the easy support on feet, or hands and feet.

3   A stationary start on the floor is followed by a travel up to and a stationary, held, curled body position on your first piece of apparatus. Pupils then stay on and travel on the apparatus, trying to emphasise changing body shapes as they go.

4   'Number one apparatus' means the group which a team brought out. Teams should be reasonable in size, and start off by standing on the floor, 3–4 metres away from their apparatus. This starting signal is matched by a similar finishing signal after including all the parts in the challenge. (Groups rotate clockwise and anti-clockwise in alternate lessons, aiming to visit three or four sets of apparatus in any one lesson. All sets of apparatus will be visited at least once per fortnight.)

Final Floor Activity

Leaping, hurdling, high bouncing, jumping, walking, hopping, hopscotch, slipping sideways.

Lesson Plan 3 • 30 minutes
November

Emphasis on: *(a) space awareness, and the unselfish sharing and good use of it (directions, levels, own and general space); (b) linking movements with obvious control and understanding.*

Floorwork
12 minutes

Legs

1   In your own small floor space, can you run with high knee-lifts? Then show me your choice of ways to travel, using legs and covering the whole floor space.

2   In your travelling all around the room, can you plan to follow the same pathway each time?

3   Can you include a direction change somewhere? Don't always travel forwards.

Body

1   Can you join together three bridge-like shapes, supporting yourself perfectly still each time on different body parts?

2   You can stand, kneel or lie, and your back, front or side can be towards the floor. You might even be up-ended on shoulders.

3   It would be very good to see two or more different levels, please. (For example, high on tiptoes, body angled down; medium crab; low sitting or lying.)

Arms

1   Can you take your body weight on to one, two or alternate hands, take your legs up into the air space above your head, then bring them down to a different floor space?

2   Handstanders can take legs high into the space. If you are happier doing lower bunny jumps, remember to plan to move your feet to a different finishing place on the floor.

3   Slow and quiet movements will look best. Keep your arm or arms straight for a safe, strong support.

Apparatus Work
16 minutes

1   Touching only the floor and mats to start with, can you show me some running or bouncing in your own floor space; include some neat, travelling actions to take you across, along, around, under, or in and out of the apparatus without touching any?

2   From a still start in a floor space each time, can you plan ways to travel up to, on to, along and from the apparatus with a change of direction somewhere?

3   Touching apparatus with hands only, take your weight onto your hands with straight arms and bent legs. Can you bring your feet down softly in a new floor space?

4   Use all the apparatus as you travel freely about the room. Plan to show me different levels at which you can travel and hold a still position on the apparatus. (For example, travel high on climbing frames; roll low across mats or pull along benches; walk in a medium crab arch; hold a high stand on a box top, a medium arch on a plank, or a low body close to a bench or mat.)

Final Floor Activity
2 minutes

Plan and show me a pattern of movements that includes an action on the spot, followed by movements where you travel forwards, sideways, backwards or diagonally.

Teaching notes and NC guidance
Development over 4 lessons

Floorwork

Legs

1 Work in your own space for about eight running steps, knees high and arms working strongly to balance legs. Then travel about the whole space, planning to make a pathway that you can remember and repeat. For example, an oval, circle, triangle or figure of eight.

2 Because pupils are following the same pathway in the whole room space, they might need to perform their travel action on the spot sometimes if they see a crowd ahead of them, impeding progress.

3 Be very careful if travelling backwards. Look over one shoulder.

Body

1 Pupils can be asked to identify any bridge-like shapes in the room as a guide to their arched shape making.

2 Demonstrations and teacher commentary on the varied possible supporting parts are necessary to increase the class repertoire. Some of the arches can be very small, such as that below knees while sitting, or below body while on elbows and knees.

3 Changing levels requires good linking movements – sitting, twisting, lowering, springing, rolling, rocking, tilting.

Arms

1 Ask class to look at a mark on the floor where they are standing at the start. Their next takeoff spot will be from a new mark.

2 Pupils can pretend to be taking weight on hands on a low box top, and coming down on the opposite side, by twisting hips and legs against the fixed hands.

3 'Slow' gives the impression of everything being under control. A still, erect starting and finishing position also enhances the appearance of the work.

Apparatus Work

1 A repeat of the starting leg activity, but with the need to plan ahead to negotiate apparatus.

2 Sideways travel on most apparatus is easy, particularly if moving on hands and feet. A jump up sideways from bench, low box or planks is done carefully and only when there is plenty of space.

3 The teacher can say 'Show me your hands and straight arms' as class hold arms forwards. Fingers should be spread and to the front, with arms in the strong, straight and safe position they will use. Short-lever, bent legs lift up more quickly than legs kept straight. On some apparatus, hands are flat on top. On others, they grip the sides. On ropes, hands are close together, gripping. On climbing frames, one hand will be gripping a bar higher than the other hand.

4 The message is probably 'on and hold; travel and hold; travel and off. Travel to next piece of apparatus.' During demonstrations the observers can be asked to 'look out for and tell me about good, held positions and their levels. Look out for and tell me about interesting travelling you see at different levels.'

Final Floor Activity

This could be as simple as a group of four jumps on the spot, alternating with jumping or travelling forwards a short distance for four, then to one side for four, then back to starting place for four.

Year 2

Lesson Plan 4 • 30 minutes
December

Emphasis on: *(a) jumping strongly and landing softly, absorbing shock; (b) rolling; (c) participating whole-heartedly in almost non-stop physical activity.*

Floorwork
12 minutes

Legs

1   Do little jumps on the spot, stretching ankles strongly to push you. Keep your body straight, but let your knees bend to make the landings soft and quiet. Jump, land, bend.

2   After a short run of about four strides, jump straight up, pushing up with one or both feet. Stretch body again in the air. Do a soft, squashy landing, with a good knee bend.

3   Now swing both arms high above head to help your jump. When you land, show me how your arms stretched forwards or sideways can help your balanced, controlled landings.

Body

1   Lie on your back, curled up small, then roll backwards and forwards from seat all the way to your shoulders and hands. Put your chin on your chest to keep your back rounded.

2   Now lie on your back, curled up small, with hands clasped under knees. Roll from side to side. Try to roll to one side, then the other side, then right over on to your back again. 'Side to side... and right over.'

3   Lie on your back with body straight and arms by your sides. Keep straight and roll over on to your front, then on to your back again. Pull across with the opposite shoulder or straight leg.

Arms

1   Put both hands on the floor with arms straight and fingers pointing forwards. Now jump your feet off the floor, gradually bouncing up higher.

2   Keep your head looking forwards. If you look back under your arms, everything will be upside down.

3   Try three or four preparatory jumps. When you feel ready, give an extra strong push to take your shoulders above your hips and your hips above your hands.

Apparatus Work
16 minutes

1   Walk around the room, touching floor and mats only. You may run and jump on to or across mats, benches and low planks.

2   When you land from your jump, try a squashy landing and a full knee bend that takes you right down on to your back. Finish by rolling sideways, spring up on to feet, and off you go again!

3   Now step up on to apparatus. Jump off, keeping your body nicely stretched, and do a soft, quiet, squashy landing. If you like, add in a sideways roll again, then off to the next apparatus.

4   Can you use a bunny-jump action to bring you on to a piece of apparatus? Hands grip sides or are flat on top, then jump and pull or twist feet up on to apparatus. Leave with either a jump, or a roll off from a sitting, kneeling or lying position.

Final Floor Activity
2 minutes

To a four-count beat, can you make up a simple pattern of jumping in your own floor space? (For example, one foot to same; one foot to other; one foot to both; both feet to both.)

Gymnastic Activities

Teaching notes and NC guidance
Development over 4 lessons

Floorwork

Legs

1   At the start, talk about and look at good ankle actions. Because the ankle joint is seldom fully extended in everyday life, there will be many poor performances. The feeling is of the head pushing up and the toes pushing and pointing down.

2   Emphasise 'upwards jump, not long jump' as pupils go higher because of the run up. Ankle and knee joints 'give' slowly on landing, to absorb shock and keep it quiet.

3   Good arm action helps the lift-off, the balance in the air, the balance on landing, and the appearance of the performance.

Body

1   We are used to travelling on feet, and on feet and hands, but not so used to travelling on other large body parts and surfaces. This long, slow rock from seat all the way to shoulders, with hands next to shoulders and thumbs in, needs to be practised and experienced. The move backwards is like the start of a backward roll. The move forwards is like the end of a forward roll.

2   Those who do not like rolling backwards and forwards do not usually mind the quite long travel of a sideways roll.

3   The straight-body sideways roll is a good rolling activity and a useful way to link two balances together.

Arms

1   For the little bounces up and down, hands are placed shoulder width apart under the shoulders, with feet and knees together.

2   Head is tilted back a little way to look ahead of where your hands are.

3   Legs are kept well bent to shorten the lever. There will be several examples of well-controlled performances in most classes. Use these to demonstrate.

Apparatus Work

1   Short runs, with the emphasis on height in the jumping when there is plenty of space and pupils are completely unimpeded.

2   With nine or ten mats available in a typical infant lesson, there will be continuous opportunities for the 'run, jump, squashy landing and roll sideways'.

3   A quick on to, up and from the apparatus, to practise landing from a greater height, with or without the sideways roll.

4   All pieces of apparatus can be arrived on by taking all the weight momentarily on the hands and doing the bunny-jump action. Pupils then travel to a point where it is possible to leave the apparatus either by a jump and a quiet landing, or by a roll.

Final Floor Activity

'Pattern' means a repeated series of actions. At least two actions are needed to make a series.

Lesson Plan 5 • 30 minutes
January

Emphasis on: *(a) sequences and linking a series of actions, and showing the ability to remember and repeat them; (b) observing performances with interest, and making comments on what was done and what was liked.*

Floorwork
12 minutes

Legs

1   Can you do an upwards jump where you are, then show me a very short run into another high jump?

2   When you are in the air, can you stretch out your body from straight arms above head down to pointed ankles and toes?

3   Be still for your start and after your finish each time. Always look for a good space to run into.

Body

1   Show me a favourite, still body shape (e.g. stretched long or wide, curled, arched, twisted). Can you move on to a different body part and show me a new body shape?

2   Make up a sequence that you can remember of three or four joined-up and changing body shapes on different body parts.

3   The linking movements will be particularly interesting to me. I will be looking for any new ideas that I can learn from (e.g. rolls, jumps, twists, lowering, rocking).

Arms

1   All start ready in a crouch position, as for a bunny jump. Show me a pattern of ways you like to travel using hands and feet. Show me contrasting actions.

2   Variety can include hands only, then feet only; walk hands, then jump feet forwards; low crawl, then high cartwheel; hands and feet wide, then close together as you travel.

3   Different body parts can lead the movements and your body can have back, front or one side towards the floor.

Apparatus Work
16 minutes

1   Show me a beautifully stretched body, standing tall on tiptoes in your own floor space. Jump on the spot, then travel up to and on to a piece of apparatus and show me a still body shape. Leave the apparatus and stop in a new floor space, nicely stretched again.

2   Start in a space near apparatus. Make your hands important in travelling up to and on to your apparatus. On the apparatus, travel using hands, or hands and feet strongly. See if some of your floorwork travelling can be used. Leave with a high jump and a nice, 'giving' landing, followed by a sideways roll if you want.

3   Starting at your number one apparatus places, try to do the following sequence for me: (a) start on the floor in your own space, do an upwards jump on the spot, then travel up to and on to the apparatus; (b) show me a firm, still body shape as soon as you arrive on your apparatus, then travel using hands, or hands and feet strongly; (c) just before leaving the apparatus, can you show me a still body shape, different from your first one; (d) leave with a stretched upwards jump or by rolling from the apparatus, and finish, still, in your own floor space.

Final Floor Activity
2 minutes

Show me a starting position with a firm, whole-body shape. Run and jump, making that shape in the air. Change your starting shape and your shape in the air.

Teaching notes and NC guidance
Development over 4 lessons

Floorwork

Legs

1 Three actions to be linked together. Jump, run and jump. The 'very short' run, of about 3 or 4 metres only, takes you into the space you decided on during your jump on the spot.

2 Twice, in the stationary and running jumps, there is an emphasis on stretching the whole body firmly to make it work as hard as possible and the actions look as good as possible.

3 Infants like to be moving all the time and need to be encouraged to hold still at start and finish.

Body

1 Arms, legs and spine work together to make the whole-body shapes. The class should be showing shapes while standing, lying, kneeling, sitting, up-ended on shoulders, arched on back or front.

2 Different body shapes on different body parts, all smoothly joined up, will be done in your own space with minimum travelling.

3 Observers can be asked to 'watch the demonstrations carefully and tell me which group of shapes you like. Tell me also how the performer linked the shapes together.'

Arms

1 Insist on slow, careful travelling, using actions that involve the whole body and put most of the weight on the hands.

2 Ask pupils to put a name to their actions, to make them think about the nature of them. (For example, crawling, hands and feet moving together; stretching out and curling in as hands only go forwards, then feet catch up; bunny jumping forwards from feet to hands, then jump feet up to hands again; bouncing on all fours as long body springs up and down, moving forwards; cartwheels.)

3 We usually travel with head leading and front of body towards the floor.

Apparatus Work

1 We are trying to encourage pupils to make a short sequence with a beginning, middle and end. This middle is simple and short – make a still body shape after arriving on the apparatus.

2 Varied travelling on hands and feet is still fresh in our memories from the floorwork. Now we practise and develop it on both floor and on apparatus, still looking for variety in actions and leading parts, and whole-body involvement.

3 If groups start at their number one apparatus places, i.e. by the piece of apparatus they brought out, the numbers will be evenly shared around all pieces. On alternate weeks pupils move around clockwise and anti-clockwise, meeting at least three sets of apparatus each lesson. The eventual demonstrations will be of whole groups showing how well they share the apparatus and floor to work almost non-stop at their sequences. They include all the elements from the training in the floorwork, here expanded and developed on floor and apparatus.

Final Floor Activity

A triangle of three actions to bring you back to your starting place is recommended.

Lesson Plan 6 • 30 minutes
February

Emphasis on: *(a) balancing; (b) maintaining good body tension and posture.*

Floorwork
12 minutes

Legs

1   Stand tall, balanced on tiptoes. Run, jump and land in a beautifully balanced position where your body is supported on one or both legs in a way that is hard to hold steady.

2   Go into your balanced finish slowly so that it becomes a landing changing into a balance, almost in slow motion.

3   The difficulty comes from being on an unusual part of one or both feet, or holding your body in a difficult position.

Body

1   Choose some part or parts of your body other than feet to balance on. Stretch those parts not being used for support to enhance the look of the balance.

2   From your first balance, can you change to a new supporting part or parts by way of a simple linking movement (such as a roll, twist, spin, arch), still not on feet?

3   Please show me your three balances nicely linked together with an interesting set of supporting parts and linking movements.

Arms

1   Swing up on to your hands and try to hold a balance for two or three seconds. Make it a strong, safe position by keeping your arms straight and your head looking forwards.

2   Try to let your swinging-up leg go a long way past your head, while the kicking foot hardly leaves the floor. A long, straight line in your legs will help to balance you.

3   'Feel' how much or how little effort is needed to take you up on to your hands. Practise and your body will remember.

Apparatus Work
16 minutes

1   As you visit each piece of apparatus, can you start off standing tall and still? Travel up to and on to the apparatus, and hold a still balance on any body part or parts. Spring up and off your apparatus with a beautifully stretched body in the air. Land in a nicely balanced position with a strong, firm body.

2   Still move from apparatus to apparatus, but this time stay longer on each piece to include travelling actions that can link up balances on different parts of the body and apparatus. Balance, travel; balance, travel; balance, travel; then spring high up and off your apparatus to land, neatly balanced.

3   Starting at your number one places, can you stay and practise to repeat, improve and remember the following: (a) start and finish on the floor in a firm, still, well-balanced position; (b) travel up to, on to, and on your apparatus, including a variety of balances on different body and apparatus parts; (c) leave apparatus with a lively spring and a well-balanced landing; and (d) have one more practice at the handstand just before your finish position.

Final Floor Activity
2 minutes

Show me the hardest balance on one or both feet that you can do without wobbling.

Teaching notes and NC guidance
Development over 4 lessons

Floorwork

Legs

1 The starting position must be a challenge to hold steady right up on tiptoes. After landing, pupils either hold a position with knees slightly bent, on tiptoes, or they move to standing on one foot, the upper body or other leg in a position that makes balancing difficult.

2 If you rush into a balance, you will almost certainly fail.

3 Near-horizontal standing on one foot, with whole body and other leg inclined forwards or to one side. Upstretched arms add to the difficulty and body tension, and improve the appearance.

Body

1 Pupils can use any body part or parts as long as there is a problem with being still. The problem is increased by the need to hold non-supporting parts stretched and firm.

2 Pupils have to plan how to move slowly to an adjacent body part to arrive in a new balance. Teacher commentary and many demonstrations will extend class repertoire of such difficult linking movements.

3 Three is sufficiently challenging, but also short enough to be remembered, practised, repeated and improved.

Arms

1 Long arms swinging from above head, or a short swing up of one leg behind you, are two controlled ways to take you on to your hands.

2 A comparison with a tightrope walker's long, straight pole is recommended to encourage a long line through both legs.

3 We are trying to develop body tension and the feeling of how much effort to apply.

Apparatus Work

1 We start off with a short, simple sequence, emphasising good, firm body tension throughout. Show a still balance at start and finish, one balance only on the apparatus, and a good move into a balance after a landing from the apparatus.

2 As in the balancing sequence in floorwork, pupils are now moving from balance to balance on apparatus, using travelling actions as linking movements.

3 Over the four weeks of the lesson's development, the class will build up their repertoire, step by step, enabling them to include all the elements within the challenge they have been given. They should experience the variety of working on three different pieces of apparatus each lesson.

Final Floor Activity

Some will make balancing difficult by working on one foot and placing the other leg in most unusual positions. Others, working on one leg, will use the whole of the upper body, placing it in such difficult positions as tilted horizontally, from upstretched arms right down to stretched, non-supporting leg.

Lesson Plan 7 • 30 minutes
March

Emphasis on: *(a) partner work, with its enjoyable and co-operative experiences; (b) working hard to achieve success.*

Floorwork
12 minutes

Legs

1 One partner practises and improves a simple, repeating floor pattern of walking, running, jumping or skipping in own floor space. The other partner practises a repeating pattern, using the whole floor space.

2 One after the other, show your sequence twice through to your partner, who watches and remembers it.

3 Can you now perform together, doing the on-the-spot pattern, then the sequence that uses the whole floor space?

Body

1 From the same starting position, facing each other, can you very slowly build up a pattern of whole-body movements, taking turns to decide the next one. I am looking for big body stretches (long and wide), curls, twists, arching.

2 Remember to work slowly so that you can mirror each other. Do two, then repeat. Improve and remember them before going on to a third movement.

3 Are you showing any variety (e.g. changing direction or level) or contrast (e.g. a sudden change of speed)?

Arms

1 Follow your leader, travelling slowly on hands and feet, repeating your pattern of three or four varied actions.

2 Leader, can you include a change of direction, not always travelling forwards?

3 Other partner, you become the new leader now. Keep working at the same sequence. Can you change it slightly by making a different body part lead (e.g. not always the head)?

Apparatus Work
16 minutes

1 One leading, one following, travel up to and on to each group of apparatus, then return to your starting place. Start again with the other partner leading, to see if he or she can remember exactly where you went and what you did.

2 This time, as you follow each other on the apparatus, try to show me good support on hands and feet, with some interesting, big body movements like you used together in the floorwork.

3 Starting on the floor on opposite sides of your piece of apparatus, can you try the following: (a) in own space, partner A demonstrates the leg activity pattern from the start of the floorwork; (b) partner B copies, then travels up to the apparatus, using one or more of the leg actions from the floorwork; (c) partner A copies the travel up to the apparatus; (d) slowly, agreeing who is leader, they pass each other, with an identical action; and (e) travel freely to finish in partner's starting position.

Final Floor Activity
2 minutes

Partner A leads a simple pattern of travelling along straight lines. Partner B leads a pattern of travelling along curving lines.

Teaching notes and NC guidance
Development over 4 lessons

Floorwork

Legs

1 They must be simple patterns, because they are to be remembered and performed, one after the other. However, to justify the name 'pattern', there must be at least two repeated actions.

2 Each watches the other, once or twice through, then they perform one after the other, starting and finishing side by side.

3 Now they 'follow the leader', facing each other for the routine on the spot, then travelling, one behind the other, using the whole room space.

Body

1 One partner leads the sequence by showing the first body action. (For example, standing with arms and legs wide, like a star.) Other partner, now in the same wide stance, leads into the second movement. (For example, lower to sitting, curled tight, head on chest.) And so on, slowly, with much repetition of first position.

2 You 'improve' by applying firm body tension to make the whole body shape look neat and under control. No slouching!

3 For example, from the curled sitting pupils could lie down and roll sideways with a stretched body on to front. A sudden change of speed can happen at the very end of a stretch or curl.

Arms

1 If the pair have their own little 'stage' to work on, not impeding others' floor space, a pattern of three or four ways to travel might take them in a triangle or rectangle back to own starting places.

2 A change of direction happens when your side or your back is leading the travelling, rather than the more usual forward-facing head.

3 Bunny jumps, for example, can be used to travel sideways, with feet and hands zig-zagging along.

Apparatus Work

1 If the travelling is kept really simple, the whole sequence can take place in instant unison, about 2 metres apart. Follower notes: What actions? How are body parts being used? What shapes are clear within the travelling? Are there any direction changes?

2 The same activity, but with a longer stay on apparatus, giving time for examples of big stretching (wide and long), curling, twisting or arching movements within your travelling.

3 Groups start at their number one apparatus places where they practise, improve and remember all the parts of their sequence. By providing good demonstrations, groups will be helped with ideas for their next piece of apparatus.

Final Floor Activity

Keep it simple enough to enable the follower to mirror the leader throughout. They change roles when the first leader stops and does an about-turn as a signal to change over duties.

Year 2

Lesson Plan 8 • 30 minutes
April

Emphasis on: *(a) awareness and good use of effort and speed to achieve a controlled performance – 'feeling' how we move; (b) using contrasting movements for a more spectacular and polished performance.*

Floorwork
12 minutes

Legs

1 Travel in a variety of ways, using legs. Can you include actions that are small, light and gentle, and actions that are large, lively and strong?

2 One way to organise it is to do the gentle actions in your own floor space, then the vigorous actions travelling away from and back to your own space.

3 Think about your actions and the ways that the feet and legs are working to make the actions 'feel' so different.

Body

1 Show me a firm balance and work hard to show a clear body shape. Being balanced means that your body has to work hard not to wobble about.

2 Contrast this strong position by relaxing and gently moving to another part or parts of the body to balance strongly again. Work your body hard to show a firm, clear shape.

3 Be strong, then relax, two or three times, as you plan your sequence of firm balances and contrasting linking actions.

Arms

1 Travel using straight arms and legs slowly and strongly, with a lot of the weight on your hands.

2 On all fours, can you experiment with hands and feet wide apart, then close together. Which is more difficult?

3 From a standing start, pretend you are travelling side to side along a bench, gripping it with hands only. Let your soft landings contrast with the strong gripping and twisting.

Apparatus Work
16 minutes

1 Travel freely all around the room, showing me easy, quiet leg actions that contrast with a strong, upwards jump on to a mat. Gentle, firm. Easy, strong. Soft, explosive.

2 Travel freely on all the apparatus. Can you contrast for me strong, firm balances, using your whole body well, and your easier travelling actions in between? Coming off, can you do a vigorous upwards jump, then a soft, 'giving' landing and gentle roll?

3 Start at your number one apparatus places to practise, repeat, improve and remember the following: (a) start and finish on the floor, away from the apparatus; (b) as you travel up to and away from the apparatus, include a change of speed at some point (e.g. an explosive jump away from the apparatus at the end of the sequence); (c) alternate travelling and balancing on the apparatus, showing strong balances and some strong travelling with arms straight.

Final Floor Activity
2 minutes

Stand still but relaxed. Accelerate into an explosive, upwards jump with an easy, gentle, quiet landing. Stand tall and relaxed. Repeat.

Teaching notes and NC guidance
Development over 4 lessons

Floorwork

Legs

1 Gentle, quiet, easy, small steps, skips and bounces. Vigorous, strong, bigger, louder galloping, running and jumping. Run with knees raising high, big bounces and long leaps from foot to foot.

2 A focus on 'where' by everyone will lead to better sharing of the floor in this space-consuming activity. They might even develop a little rhythm. On the spot, 3, 4, 5, 6; travelling for 1... and 2... and 3... and 4... and 5... and home again!

3 To be able to demonstrate ('Who will volunteer?'), pupils must know their actions and uses of the relevant body parts.

Body

1 Ensure that pupils are balancing with difficulty and not just standing, kneeling or sitting easily.

2 From 'feeling strong' in their firm balance, ask them to feel relaxed and easy as they transfer to another supporting body part, then firm up strongly again.

3 An obvious contrast is in the use of levels, from highest position on tiptoes or one foot, down to being on one knee and one elbow, for example.

Arms

1 On all fours, walking action; hands only, then feet only; front or back towards floor; hands walk, feet jump to astride hands; or cartwheels.

2 Wide is difficult because arms are at an angle. Close is difficult because you need to be supple enough to bring feet near to hands, arching high.

3 All weight on hands will happen more often now, e.g. for the vertical or lower than vertical cartwheels, or the swing of legs across while staying on hands.

Apparatus Work

1 The quiet, easy actions will be slower than the accelerating sprint into the dynamic jump.

2 On the apparatus, strong, still balances will alternate two or three times with travelling. At any one time, the hall should be full of still, strong, firm balances and travelling. If necessary, to reinforce the inclusion of balances, the teacher can call out 'Be still, those who are now balancing. The others, keep on travelling, and now... stop! Balancers, start your turn to travel now, keep going... and stop!'

3 All the elements from the floorwork are now being asked for on both floor and apparatus. There will be contrasts of speed and effort, and different 'feelings' within the bodies of the performers at the different parts of their sequences.

Final Floor Activity

As pupils stand still and tall, their weight is slightly forwards on the balls of the feet, ready for the off. From stillness, they burst into acceleration for the jump, with its explosive drive up and off. A quiet landing nearly in slow motion, with knees and ankles 'giving' and often one foot landing after the other, provides contrasting leg activity.

Year 2

Lesson Plan 9 • 30 minutes
May

Emphasis on: *(a) sequences and working harder for longer; (b) responding to set tasks with enthusiasm and confidence.*

Floorwork
12 minutes

Legs

1 Using your legs, show me a triangle of movements, starting and finishing at the same place. Can you include three different actions and be aware of your body shapes?

2 Variety will come from your different actions and directions. Contrast can come from a change of speed or effort at some point. (An easy, slow, gentle action contrasts with a vigorous, accelerating one.)

3 Legs can travel down at floor level, and lift up higher in shapes like a hurdler, star, tuck, jack-knife, or a mixture (e.g. one leg straight down, the other bent back).

Body

1 Practise backward, forward and side-to-side rolls from a curled-up sitting position. When you go backwards and forwards, put your hands next to your shoulders and push forwards with them. Side to side, keep hands clasped under knees.

2 Try to roll to one side, to other side, to first side and right over on to your back again. Side, side, side and over.

3 Lie on your back with arms by your side. Twist by lifting one shoulder or leg to take you into a sideways roll, on to front and on to back again.

4 Now, you choose. Start from a low crouch position; or sitting curled; or lying stretched, and plan a roll sequence to include at least two of the three we have practised.

Arms

1 Slowly and quietly, show me two or more ways to travel on hands, or hands and feet, and see if you could give each action a name, as an introduction, if I asked you to demonstrate.

2 Work in your own small floor space, and show me a still position to signal start and finish each time.

3 Variety will come from a good mixture, such as high on hands, walking or cartwheeling; medium on strong, straight arms and legs, sometimes legs only, sometimes arms only; and low, crouched bunny-jump actions on hands, with bent legs doing a variety of movements.

Apparatus Work
16 minutes

1 Visit each set of apparatus in turn and show me a different method of travelling up to and on to each one for a very short time. Then travel away to a new floor space for your next, different travel.

2 Continue to travel to the apparatus in different ways, but this time take all the weight on your hands to bring you on to the apparatus. A strong bunny-jump grip and action should work at most pieces. Leave with a high jump, a squashy landing and, if there is space on your mat, try a roll.

3 Starting at your number one apparatus places, can you practise, repeat, improve and remember a short sequence of your favourite activities on that apparatus and surrounding floor space?

Final Floor Activity
2 minutes

In a running sequence, can you include changes of direction, body shape and speed?

Teaching notes and NC guidance
Development over 4 lessons

Floorwork

Legs

1. Ask the class to walk around their little triangle with its 3-metre sides, starting and finishing on the same mark, line, floorboard (or whatever) each time. Walking might even be one of their three different actions.

2. 'Different actions' infers greatly differing uses of feet and legs. (For example, easy passing each other as in walking; vigorous running into a leap; hopscotch; mixture of actions.)

3. Asking for 'low, middling and higher feet and leg actions' should inspire some varied ideas worth demonstrating.

Body

1. The 'hands beside shoulders, thumbs in and fingers spread' is an important teaching point. In a backward roll, hands at shoulders push you on to feet. In a forward roll, hands push you forwards and up on to feet.

2. In rolling sideways, a swing into the movement by the combined knees and clasped hands is essential for a lively action.

3. Left shoulder or leg does the twisting pull to the right.

4. For example, from a low crouch, lower to sitting, and rock backwards and forwards; roll side to side and over on to back; stretch out straight lying on back; roll to left, then to right; sit up curled, rock back on to shoulders and hands; push forwards strongly up on to feet and back to starting crouch position.

Arms

1. For example, 'I am crawling with straight arms and legs; then walking hands only forwards, and jumping feet up to hands; then I finish with a cartwheel.'

2. If you are kicking feet up to go on to hands, always check that you have room behind you, away from others or apparatus.

3. Like direction changes, level changes provide an obvious and interesting contrast within a performance.

Apparatus Work

1. The 'up to and away from' travelling is the main emphasis. The two different methods of travel can use feet, or feet and hands.

2. 'Feel strong in your hands and arms as you lift, pull, twist, roll, lever, spring' on to apparatus. For variety there should be a strong leg action into the upwards jump and landing, and an easy, slow roll on a mat.

3. During this relatively free activity, the teacher will be able to assess how well the class work on and share the floor and apparatus space; how confident and competent they are in managing their bodies in a wide range of apparatus situations; and how enthusiastically and whole-heartedly they participate in their vigorous physical activity.

Final Floor Activity

Changing speed in their running will include running on the spot when their progress is impeded by others, plus slowing down and speeding up. Go backwards with great care, looking over one shoulder.

Year 2

Lesson Plan 10 • 30 minutes
June

Emphasis on: *(a) partner work to provide enjoyable new learning and social experiences not possible on one's own; (b) extending movement understanding because you need to recognise your partner's movements and be able to repeat your own.*

Floorwork
12 minutes

Legs

1 Travel side by side or follow the leader, going from space to space. Plan and agree the three varied actions you will use, i.e. one easy and quiet, one with a direction change, and one that explodes into a vigorous movement.

2 Start and finish standing still. After your third movement, go again when you see a big enough space for two of you.

3 A mixture of leading and following, and side by side, would be very interesting (e.g. side by side, going sideways).

Body

1 Start off, not on your feet, and curl up very small. Stretch part of your body to reach out into the space around you. Curl in tight to support yourself on a new body part.

2 Stretch a different part of your body to a different place in the surrounding space. Curl in tight to your first supporting body part.

3 Show each other your curls and stretches. Plan a way to perform them together, with some contact between you on the two stretches. (Partners will need to adjust their starting positions and relationships to accommodate the stretches.)

Arms

1 Partner A demonstrates a favourite way to travel on feet and hands, or to be supported on hands only. Partner B observes.

2 Partner B repeats this first action, and adds on one of his or her favourites. Partner A watches.

3 Partner A repeats the two actions, and adds on a third one. Partner B watches carefully.

4 Partner B performs all three actions only or adds in a fourth and last action, with partner A's approval.

Apparatus Work
16 minutes

1 Follow your leader, who travels a short distance on floor and apparatus then stops, to let you copy and catch up. I would like to see some of the varied actions we did on the floor earlier.

2 On apparatus, I would like to see the new leader demonstrating ways to go from a tight curl to a full stretch with a body part reaching out into space. Partner, once again, will observe, then copy. Travel freely, from apparatus to apparatus.

3 Starting at your number one apparatus places, plan and practise: (a) a still starting position on the floor, one behind the other; (b) follow the leader, travelling up to and on to apparatus, using hands strongly to support you, then hold a tight curled position next to each other. New leader takes over, leads slowly into a full stretch, and then travels on apparatus, using hands and feet; (c) same leader comes away from apparatus, using a different leg action from the one that took you on at start.

Final Floor Activity
2 minutes

Take it in turns to be leader. Jump on the spot, then run and jump to face a new direction.

Teaching notes and NC guidance
Development over 4 lessons

Floorwork

Legs

1 Travelling on a diagonal, one slightly behind the other, takes little space, and still lets one observe the other. Recommend all travel in a straight line, not anti-clockwise in a big circle, getting in one another's way, as so often happens in primary schools.

2 'Your movement is like a sentence, with a start and a finish each time, please.' (A 'sentence' of three words.)

3 Pupils can be very creative and include: one working on the spot, one circling; or parting and closing as they travel.

Body

1 In the 'stretching and curling sequence', the stretching parts are varied and reach out into different places in space. (Can be to front, side, rear, low, high.) To enable this, we change our starting positions.

2 They can be asked to 'feel' strong and firm as they stretch out the whole body. (No sagging!) Then they 'feel' relaxed and gentle as they fold in to their contrasting curl.

3 Partners can be back to back; side by side; side to back; or facing, as necessary, to permit the momentary contact in the stretches.

Arms

1 'One favourite way only' must be emphasised, and we want the new activity to be within the capability of the observer.

2 The second action needs to be able to flow on from the first, without too much of a linking problem.

3 As well as being easily linked, we want the next action to have something different about it to maintain the performers' and (later) observers' interest. 'Different' may be the change of level, direction, body shape, body part leading or towards floor, and, of course, actions.

4 The three or four activities, all flowing one after the other, should take three or four lessons to decide and develop.

Apparatus Work

1 Leader goes and stops while partner observes the actions and any changes of direction, shape or speed. Following partner catches up with leader and stops. Leader, alone, goes and stops.

2 If space permits on a piece of apparatus, include two or three examples of curling, then stretching. On mats, this can include rolls into kneeling, lying or standing stretched. On mats, benches, planks or low box top, the curl can be crouched on two feet, lying on back, front or one side, on knees, up-ended on shoulder and hands. Follow these with the many possible stretchings out.

3 The various floorwork activities are now requested, this time to be performed on floor and apparatus. Include: (a) two ways to travel between apparatus and starting/finishing place on floor; (b) taking whole body weight on hands, and travelling using hands and feet; (c) curling and stretching; (d) observing, copying and working in unison with a partner.

Final Floor Activity

On the 'jump to face a new direction', partners can arrange to change over their roles as leader and follower.

Lesson Plan 11 • 30 minutes
July

Emphasis on: *(a) planning activities safely, and performing them with control; (b) practising whole-heartedly to improve, alone and with others; (c) reflecting and commenting on what they and others have done.*

Floorwork
12 minutes

Legs

1 Rise up on tiptoes with arms nicely stretched sideways for balance. Walk, then run a short distance to jump high and land facing a new direction. Let arms help balance.

2 Each time, look for a clear space, and plan where you will go for your next jump. Never disturb others in the room.

3 Changing direction is helped in the air if you swing into your jump with a strong arm or leg action. Or you can change direction on or after landing.

Body

1 Make a bridge-like shape, standing with feet apart, body arched forwards, arms angled to the floor. Show me that you can make a different body shape. (For example, feet together, bend legs and back to go down to a curled shape.)

2 Can you now change to a new bridge-like shape? (For example, sitting with bridge below knees.)

3 In your own space, continue to change from a bridge to another shape, back to a bridge, then to another shape. A sequence of three of each would be pleasing.

Arms

1 Show a partner your best way to take your body weight onto your hands. Your partner will watch, then tell you what he or she particularly liked about your demonstration.

2 Change over. Now the other partner shows a favourite way to take all the weight on to the hands. Once again, the watcher tells what was liked in the demonstration.

3 You might like the neat, still, starting and finishing position; the good, safe, straight arms; the neat body shape, maybe with legs straight and together; or the nice high hips in a bunny jump. Say what you liked.

Apparatus Work
16 minutes

1 Follow your partner, who will take you up to each piece of apparatus, show you a way to take weight onto hands only on the apparatus, then move on to the next place. On and off quickly.

2 Other partner now leads, and shows a short walk, a short run and a careful jump to land on a mat or to cross mat, bench, low plank or low box top. When you land you can try a squashy landing and a roll if you like. Following partner stays back, watching, until there is space to follow and copy.

3 On your own now, start at your number one apparatus places to practise, repeat, improve and remember: (a) a still start and finish on the floor, away from apparatus; (b) travelling on to apparatus, using your arms strongly as you move along or support yourself; (c) within your travelling to see how often you can make a bridge-like shape on apparatus, or on apparatus and adjacent floor.

Final Floor Activity
2 minutes

Stand, balanced, on one or parts of both feet, with arms stretched. Walk a few steps and stop in a different balance on one or both feet.

Teaching notes and NC guidance
Development over 4 lessons

Floorwork

Legs

1 This activity needs a lot of whole-body control and good body tension as you hold a balanced start; run and jump to land steady without a stumble or wobble; and organise your direction change.

2 The runs must never be long because the run and jump are of equal importance. Some runs might only need two or three strides if the only space is nearby.

3 A swing up with one arm or leg turns your body towards the other side, often helpful if you are approaching a wall.

Body

1 The nature of a 'bridge-like shape' can be emphasised by asking the class to point out examples in the hall, to identify the arched shape.

2 Bridges can be held standing with front, back or one side towards the floor; or up-ended on shoulders, head and hands.

3 Variety comes from different supporting parts and different levels. (For example, high on feet; medium on one hand and one foot with one side towards floor; low on heels and shoulders, back towards floor.)

Arms

1 All weight has to be supported on hands for a second or two. Many will do cartwheels and handstands. Others will do a bunny jump.

2 Each can demonstrate two or three times to ensure at least one good one.

3 'Reflecting and evaluating' is a requirement within National Curriculum Physical Education. Working in pairs enables every pupil to practise this skill without the possible embarrassment of speaking to the whole class.

Apparatus Work

1 Because this is a simple activity, partners can follow quite close, one behind the other. 'On how many apparatus surfaces can you and your partner perform, with straight arms and bent legs, in the next minute?'

2 Leading partner is responsible for planning to go where both partners will have space to perform the approach, the jump, and the landing and roll.

3 About five minutes are spent practising at each of the three sets of apparatus they will try to visit. This gives time to practise, repeat and improve their sequences. The emphasis is on strong arm support as you travel, alternating with stops at various places to demonstrate a still, bridge-like shape. The still, erect start and finish should be pursued as a way for the performer to signal 'I am ready to start' and 'I have completed my sequence'.

Final Floor Activity

If a still balance on one foot is beyond anyone's ability, tell them to place the toes of the other foot on the floor to help balance. The balances can be 'different' by holding non-supporting foot in different ways, or by inclining the upper body in different ways, e.g. horizontally forwards, to side, or back.

Dance

The Aims of Dance

Education has been described as the 'structuring of experiences in such a way as to bring about an increase in human capacity'. Dance aims to increase human capacity under the following headings:

1 **Physical development**. We focus on body action to develop skilful, well-controlled, versatile movement. We want our pupils to move well, looking poised and confident. The vigorous actions in dance also promote healthy physical development, fitness and strength.

2 **Knowledge and understanding**. Pupils learn and understand through the combination of physical activity (with its doing, feeling and experiencing of movement) and the mental processes of decision-making, as they plan, refine, evaluate and then plan again for improvement.

3 **Enjoyment**. Dance is fun and an interesting, sociable, enjoyable physical activity. In addition to the perspiration and deep breathing which the vigorous physical activity inspires, there should be smiling faces expressing enjoyment. When asked why they like something, pupils' first answer is usually 'It's fun!' It is hoped that enjoyable, sociable and physical activity experienced regularly at school in dance and other physical education lessons, can have an influence on pupils' eventual choice of lifestyle, long after they have left school. We want them to understand that regular physical activity makes you look and feel better, and helps to make you feel relaxed, calm and fit.

4 **Confidence and self-esteem**. Particularly at primary school, a good physical education that recognises and praises achievement can enhance an individual's regard for him or herself, and help to improve confidence and self-esteem. Dance lessons are extremely visual and offer many opportunities to see improvement, success and creativity; demonstrating these admirable achievements to others; and helping pupils feel good about themselves.

5 **Social development**. Friendly, co-operative social relationships are part of most dance lessons. Achievement, particularly in the 'dance climax' part of the lesson, is usually shared with a partner or a small group. Pupils also share space sensibly with others; take turns at working; demonstrate to, and watch demonstrations by, others; and make appreciative, helpful comments to demonstrators and partners.

6 **Creativity**. It has been said that 'if you have never created something, you have never experienced satisfaction.' Dance is a most satisfying activity, regularly challenging pupils to plan and present something original. Opportunities abound for an appreciative teacher to say 'Thank you for your demonstration and your own, original way of doing the movements.'

7 **Expression and Communication**. In dance we communicate through the expression in movement of the feelings or the action. We use, for example, stamping feet to express anger; we skip, punch the air or clap hands to show happiness; we swagger, head held high, to express self-assurance. Similarly, we create simple characters and stories by expressing them through movements associated with them. The old or young; machine or leaves; puppet, animal or circus clown, can all be expressed through their particular way of moving.

8 **Artistic and aesthetic appreciation**. Gaining knowledge and understanding of the quality-enhancing elements of movement is a particular aim of dance. Such understanding of quality, variety and contrast in the use of body action, shape, direction, size, speed and force, is a major contributor to appreciation of good movement. We want our pupils to understand what is good about good movement.

Teaching Dance

Dance might appear to be the easiest physical education subject to teach because there are no elusive and unpredictable implements hampering a lesson's flow as in games, and there is no large apparatus to lift, carry, place and use safely and sensibly, as in gymnastic activities.

In fact, dance is the hardest subject to teach because a dance lesson needs the constant involvement of the teacher. A popular game can keep a class busy for long periods with little teacher input, while apparatus work in gymnastic activities inspires so many exciting, challenging actions that pupils can be kept busy, even if the teacher has little to say.

This 'ongoing potential' for minimum teacher involvement does not apply in dance. A dance, once completed and presented, does not have the prolonged 'shelf life' of a game or apparatus work.

We do not always need a story or a big theme as a starting point. Action words called out by the teacher, or seen on a card, can almost instantly get the class working because the task is specific. Any creative development requested should be equally clear, for example, 'Make a short sequence, using skip, stretch and turn in any order you choose.'

Everyone can use their imagination but they need to be clear about what they are being asked to do and when to do it, when challenged to create more expressive sequences and patterns. Guidance must be specific. The teacher's difficult task is to remove all vagueness and give the class an easily visualised, clearly understood image, so that they know exactly what they are being asked to do.

If pupils are set vague tasks such as 'Find ways...', 'Make shapes...', or 'Explore levels...', they will not understand why they are finding, making or exploring, because there is no obvious end to it. Such a task is not specific enough and does not conjure up an easily visualised image. Doing 'creeping and crawling' is much more purposeful if we are moving like a burglar about to enter a house. Balancing like a tightrope walker is much more interesting than being told to 'Travel slowly along a straight line.' Within the theme 'Nature', 'Explore being a butterfly' is too loose and vague. Instead, we can look at the life cycle of the butterfly:

a in the egg – all curled up as individuals,

b the wiggling up and down of the caterpillar,

c into the fluttering, flying butterfly, which can be represented by one or more dancers, and then

d it dies.

The dance has been given form and structure. Teacher and class have a clear picture in their heads; they know what to do; and they know where the dance is going.

Stimuli as Starting Points with which to Inspire Dance Action

Stimuli are used to gain the interest of the class, provide a focus for their attention, get them into the action quickly, and inspire in them a desire for movement.

A dance stimulus is something you:

○ **enjoy doing**, such as natural actions. Pupils will immediately start to walk, run, jump, skip, hop, bounce or gallop, whether accompanied by music, percussion, following the teacher/leader, or responding to an enthusiastic teacher calling out the actions.

○ **can hear**. Sounds that stimulate movement include:

   a   medium to quick tempo music, including folk dance music

   b   percussion instruments – tambourine, drum, cymbal, clappers

   c   body contact sounds – clapping hands, stamping feet, slapping body, clicking fingers

   d   rhythmically chanted phrases, words, place names or actions which can be shortened or elongated to inspire and accompany actions

   e   vocal sounds to accompany actions, on the spot and travelling as in 'toom, toom, toom' marching; 'boomp, boomp, boomp' bouncing; and 'tick, tock, tick, tock' slow stepping

   f   action songs, chanted rhymes and nursery rhymes.

○ **can see or imagine**. Objects like a leaf, branch, balloon, ball, bubble, puppet, rag doll, firework, can all be used to suggest movement ideas to children. Use of imagery and imagination helps to communicate what we are trying to express more clearly. 'Can you creep softly and slowly, as if you did not want to be heard, coming home late?'

○ **have seen on a visit, on television, or in a photograph**. Of particular interest to pupils are:

   a   zoo animals – penguins. elephants, dolphins, monkeys

   b   circus performers – jugglers, clowns, trapeze artists, acrobats, tightrope walkers

   c   seaside play – swimming, paddling, making sandcastles, plus movements of the waves

   d   children's playground activities – climbing, swinging, sea-saw, throwing and catching, skipping, circling on a roundabout.

○ **experience seasonally** – spring and growth, summer holidays, autumn and harvest, winter snow and frost, Guy Fawkes' Night, Halloween, Christmas toys, circus and pantomime, Easter eggs.

○ **consider newsworthy or of human interest** – Olympic Games, extremes of weather, newly arrived pupils, hobbies, family, friendship, approaching holidays.

Whatever the starting point, the teacher must convert it into the language of movement. Children cannot 'be' leaves, but they can 'Travel on tip toes with light, floating movements, tilting and turning slowly.' They cannot 'be' clowns, but they can 'Do a funny walk on heels, spin round with one leg high, fall down slowly, bounce up and repeat.' They cannot 'be' machines, but they can 'Try pushing down actions, like corks into bottles, on the spot, turning or moving along, as on an assembly line.'

The Creative Dance Lesson Plan

Warming up Activities which start the lesson are important because they can create an attentive, co-operative, industrious and thoughtful start to the lesson, put the class in the mood for dance, and encourage them to move with good body poise and tension, sharing the floor unselfishly. The activities need to be simple enough to get the whole class working, almost immediately, often by following the teacher who, ideally, is a stimulating **'purveyor of action'** enthusiastically leading the whole class, often by example, into wholehearted participation in simple activities which need little explanation. Some form of travelling, using the feet, is often the warming-up activity, with a specific way of moving being asked for. It might be to show better use of space, greater variety, greater control, good poise and body tension, or simply an enthusiastic use of all the body parts to warm up.

The Movement Skills Training middle part of the lesson is used to teach and develop the movement skills and patterns that are to be used in the new dance. Here, the teacher is an **educator**, informing, challenging, questioning, using demonstrations and sometimes direct teaching.

a Kneel down and curl to your smallest shape. Show me how you can start to grow, very slowly. Are you starting with your back, head, shoulders, elbows or arms? Show me clearly how you rise to a full, wide stretch position.

b If gesturing is like speaking with your body's movement, how might your body gesture say 'I am angry'? Stamp feet, clench fists, punch the air, jump up and down heavily.

c How are bubbles (made by teacher and pupils) moving? Where are they going? Floating gently, gliding smoothly, soaring from low to higher, sinking slowly.

The creating and performing Dance Climax of the lesson is the most important part and must not be missed out or rushed. If necessary, earlier parts of the lesson should be reduced. Here the teacher is a **coach**, helping and guiding the pupils as they work at their creation, moving round to all parts of the room to advise, encourage, enthuse, praise and, eventually, demonstrate.

a Slowly, start to grow and show me which parts are leading as you rise to your full, wide flower shape in our 'Spring Dance'. You might even twist your flower shape to look at the sun.

b Find a partner for our 'Gestures' dance and decide who is asking a favour by gesturing with body actions to say 'Please! I'm desperate! I need it! I must have it!' The other partner's body actions are saying 'Never! You must be joking! Go away!' When we look at demonstrations later, we will decide who the most expressive winners are.

c For our 'Bubbles dance', I will say the four actions that are to be practised – floating gently, gliding smoothly, soaring, sinking slowly, and you will show me how you have planned to dance them.

Depending on its complexity, a dance lesson will be repeated three or four times to allow sufficient time for repetition, practice and improvement to take place, and a satisfactory performance to be achieved and presented.

It has been said that 'dance is all about making, remembering and repeating patterns.' Whether we are performing a created dance or an existing folk dance, there will still be a still start and finish, and an arrangement of repeated parts within.

The Traditional Folk Dance Lesson Plan – 30 minutes

Warming-up Activities – 5 minutes

These varied steps can relate to the new figures to be taught, or they can be travelling steps or steps on the spot of any kind, to stimulate quick, easy enjoyable action to put the class in the mood for dance. The warm-up can be done alone or with a partner. As well as inspiring action, the teacher establishes high standards of neat footwork and good, safe, unselfish sharing of space. For example, 'Skip by yourself, to visit all parts of the room, keeping in time with the music.' 'When drum sounds twice, join hands with the nearest person and dance together.' 'When drum sounds once, dance by yourself again.'

Teach Figures of New Dance – 14 minutes

Teaching is easier in a big circle formation where everyone can see and copy the teacher. Often, all can perform the whole dance together, slowly and carefully, figure by figure, practising it to the teacher's voice, then doing it at the correct speed. The teacher's non-stop vocal accompaniment, along with the actions, serves to remind the class of the actions and keeps them moving at the correct speed. For example, 'Everyone ready... Skip to the centre, 2, 3, turn on 4; back to places, 2, 3, arrive on 4. Boys to centre, 2, 3, turn on 4; back to places, 2, 3, there on 4. Girls to centre, 2, 3, turn on 4; back to places, 2, 3, hands joined on 4. All circle left, 2, 3, 4, 5, 6, back the other way; circle right, 2, 3, 4, 5, 6, ready to start again.'

Teaching in sets of two, three, four or more couples is more difficult because the sets are separate, with someone's back to the teacher. Each leading couple in turn will be taken slowly through the figures, then walking, then dancing to the music or the teacher's vocal accompaniment.

Teach the New Dance – 7 minutes

Ideally, the new dance will be performed without stopping, helped by early reminders to the next dancers from the teacher's continuous vocal accompaniment. It is sometimes necessary to stop the music after each dancing couple has completed the dance, because of problems experienced by some of the dancers. The new couples are put in position, the music is re-started, and they do the dance once again.

Revise a Favourite Dance – 4 minutes

This last dance, often chosen by pupils, should be a contrast to the lesson's new dance, for variety. A lively circle dance, with all dancing non-stop, can be contrasted with a set dance where only one or two of the four couples are dancing at a time.

Teaching Dance with 'Pace'

High on the list of accolades for an excellent dance lesson is the comment that 'it had excellent pace' and moved along, almost non-stop, from start to finish. Lesson pace is determined by the way that each of the several skills making up the whole lesson is taught. For example:

1 **Quickly into action**. Using few words, explain the skill clearly and challenge the class to begin. 'Show me your best stepping, in time with the music. Begin!' This near-instant start is helped if the teacher joins in and works enthusiastically with them.

2 **Emphasise the main teaching points, one at a time, while class is working**. The class all need to be working quietly if the teacher is to be heard. 'Visit all parts of the room – sides, ends and corners, as well as the middle.' 'Travel along straight lines, never following anyone.' (Primary school pupils always travel in a big anti-clockwise circle, all following one another, unless taught otherwise.)

3 **Identify and praise good work while the class is working**. The class teacher does not say 'well done' without being specific and explaining what is praiseworthy. Comments are heard by all and remind the class of key points. 'Well done, Emily. Your tiptoe stepping is lively and neat.' 'Daniel, you keep finding good spaces to travel through. Well done.'

4 **Teach for individual improvement, while the class is working**. 'Michael, swing arms and legs with more determination, please.' 'Rachel, use your eyes each time you change direction to see where the best space is.'

5 **Use a demonstration, briefly**, to show good quality, or a good example of what is expected and worth copying. 'Stop, please, and watch Sophie, Michael, James and Chloe step out firmly with neat, quiet footwork, never following anyone.' 'Stop and watch how Ellie is mixing bent, straight and swinging leg actions for variety.'

6 **Very occasionally, to avoid using too much activity time, a short demonstration is followed by comments from observers**. 'Half of the class will watch the other half. Look out for and tell me whose stepping is neat, lively and always well spaced. Tell me if someone impresses you for any other reason.' The class watch for about 12 seconds and three or four comments are listened to. For example: 'John is mixing tiny steps with big ones.' 'Sophie is stepping with feet passing each other, then with feet wide apart.' Halves of the class change over and repeat the demonstrations with comments.

7 **Thanks are given to all the performers and to those who made helpful, friendly comments**. Further practice takes place with reminders of the good things seen and commented on.

A Pattern For Looking at and Developing Dance Movement

To avoid confusing him or herself and the class, the teacher will be thinking about, looking for and talking about one element within dance at a time. If, in the early stages of a lesson's development, the teacher is only looking for the actions and how the body parts concerned are performing them, there is some hope for progress and improvement. If, on the other hand, the teacher is exhorting the class to think about 'your spacing, actions, shape, speed – and what about some direction changes?', all at the same time, then confusion will be the only outcome.

Stage 1 The Body

What is the pupil doing?

1	**Actions**	travelling, jumping, turning, rolling, balancing, gesturing, rising, falling, etc.
2	**Body parts**	legs, feet, hands, shoulders, head, etc.
3	**Body shape**	stretched, curled, wide. twisted, arched.

Stage 2 The Space

Where is the pupil doing it?

1	**Directions**	forwards, backwards, sideways.
2	**Level**	high, medium, low.
3	**Size**	own, little, personal space; whole room, large general space shared with others.

CHILD

DANCING

Stage 3 The Quality

How is the pupil doing it?

1	**Weight or effort**	firm, gentle, vigorous, light, heavy.
2	**Time or speed**	sudden, fat, slow, speeding up, slowing down, explosive.

Stage 4 The Relationships

With whom is the pupil doing it?

1	**Alone**	but always conscious of sharing space with others.
2	**Teacher**	near, following, mirroring, in circle with, away from, towards.
3	**Partner**	leading, following, meeting, parting, mirroring, copying, making contact with.
4	**Group**	circle, part of class for a demonstration.

Stages in Creating and Progressing a Dance

First of all, decide what the dance will be about. For example, autumn leaves, making a puppet, or fireworks.

Stage 1
Decide which actions, neatly performed, will be used to represent the subject and to express it in movement.

Autumn leaves hover, float, glide, rise, fall, tilt and turn, then sink to the ground. The whole body makes the leaf shape, which may have parts curling in, sticking out, both smooth and crinkly. Puppets move in a floppy, loose way, as if they have no muscles, only bones that move jerkily as if pulled by strings. The puppet's arms can bend, swing, circle or reach up into a long or wide, stretched shape. Fireworks include rockets whooshing into flight, sparklers sending out their sparks, and bangers jumping noisily and unexpectedly. The arms can reach forwards to make a rocket shape.

Decide how best to use body parts and shapes to make the actions look poised, neat, correct and well-controlled.

The whole body makes the shape of autumn leaves which include parts curling in, parts sticking out, some smooth, some crinkly. The puppet's arms can lift jerkily and alternately, as if pulled up straight by strings, then drop to bend and flop again. The rocket is represented by both arms reaching forward to make a long streamlined shape.

Stage 2
Decide how to use the whole room space, as if it is a stage, to make the dance more interesting and exciting.

Autumn leaves soar from low to high, turn in the same space, hover, hardly moving, glide to a far corner, drop to the ground, straight or with a spiralling action. Puppets, learning how to move, experiment by using the hands and arms to reach out into space in front, to the sides, behind and overhead. Fireworks are interesting with the contrasting actions of the rocket's straight whoosh, the Catherine wheel's spinning, and the unpredictable jumping and shifting of the bangers.

Stage 3
Consider how the performance might be made more attractive, surprising and expressive by applying just the right amount of **speed and force**.

The slow and gentle rise and fall of autumn leaves, still attached to their branches, contrasts with the sudden, almost explosive snap and break away from the branch. Puppets can circle their arms gently and slowly, and then punch the air firmly and strongly. With fireworks, the long, smooth, ongoing rocket zoom contrasts with its eventual sudden, explosive, fragmented scattering.

Stage 4
With whom are we dancing? What are our relationships with the others in the room?

Even if 'Autumn Leaves' is an individual dance, we share the floor space unselfishly with others as we weave, swoop, soar, hover, glide, tilt and turn, in and out, alongside or around them. In 'Puppet Makers' the puppet and the maker mirror each other in learning to move, and in leading and following. In a 'Fireworks' dance, the pupils start, one group at a time. 'Sparklers, begin! Bangers get ready, begin! Sparklers, keep going! Rockets, ready... go! Sparklers, bangers, rockets, all stop now.' They all can combine to flicker and sparkle in the bonfire, interweaving, shooting, crackling, subsiding, dying.

Headings when Considering a Pupil's Achievement and Progress through Dance

Physical fitness

Strong, often prolonged physical activity, inspired by vigorous leg action, helps to promote normal, healthy growth and physical development. Lively leg action in dance also stimulates strong heart and lungs activity, leading to improved stamina.

Physical skill and versatility

Body management and self-control, called for in challenging situations, develops skill in natural actions such as travelling, jumping and landing, balancing, rolling, turning, rising and falling. When body management and self-control are good, there is an impression of poised, confident, versatile, safe movement.

Feeling valued and self-confident

Using their imagination, being creative, planning something original, and then sharing it with others, can develop and improve pupils' self confidence and self-esteem, particularly when the teacher and the class warmly and enthusiastically express their appreciation for the achievement. We want our dancers, eventually, to exude confidence and enthusiasm.

Expressing themselves

Using the body as an instrument of expression, and another way to communicate, pupils can express emotions, inner feelings, moods, convey ideas, and even create simple characters and stories. For many, this is a totally different, potentially eloquent outlet for expressing feeling as they stamp the work with their own personality.

Learning to develop friendly, co-operative, working relationships with others

Dance is the most sociable of physical education's activities. Working in pairs and groups; sharing space; taking turns; demonstrating and being demonstrated to; and appreciating and being appreciated by others, encourages desirable, enjoyable, co-operative social relationships.

Believing in the value of participation in physical activity

We want pupils to look and feel better after exercise, and believe that physical activity is enjoyable, and an essential antidote to the increasingly sedentary, inactive lifestyle of many people.

Becoming more competent, knowledgeable performers and spectators

Dance education develops an appreciation of the aesthetic and expressive elements within dance – variety and contrast in actions, shape, direction and level, speed, and degree of force.

National Curriculum Requirements for Dance – Key Stage 1: the Main Features

'The government believes that two hours of physical activity a week, including the National Curriculum for Physical Education and extra-curricular activities, should be an aspiration for all schools. This applies to all key stages.'

Programme of study
Pupils should be taught to:

a use movement imaginatively, responding to stimuli, including music, and performing basic skills (e.g. travelling, being still, making a shape, jumping, turning, gesturing)
b change the rhythm, speed, level and direction of their movements
c create and perform dances using simple movement patterns, including those from different times and cultures
d express and communicate ideas and feelings.

Attainment targets
Pupils should be able to demonstrate that they can:

a select and use skills, actions and ideas appropriately, applying them with co-ordination and control
b copy, explore, repeat and remember skills, and link them in ways that suit the activities
c talk about differences between their own and others' work; suggest improvements; and use this understanding to improve their performance.

Main NC headings when considering assessment, progression and expectation

Planning – mostly before performing, but planning also takes place during performance, with pupils making quick decisions to find a space or adapt a skill. In these initial, exploratory stages, pupils try things out and learn from early efforts. When planning is satisfactory, there is evidence of a clear understanding of the task; good use of own ideas; good judgements being made; and consideration for others sharing the space.

Performing and improving performance – always the main outcome to be achieved and we are fortunate that the visual nature of Physical Education enables pupils' achievements to be easily seen and judged. When performing is satisfactory, there is evidence of well-controlled, thoughtful, neat, safe and successful outcomes; originality, versatility and a capacity for almost non-stop work, alone and with others; simple skills being performed accurately and linked together with increasing control and consistency and the ability to repeat and remember.

Linking actions – pupils build longer, 'joined-up' sequences of linked actions in response to the task set and stimuli used. In the same way that joined-up words make language and joined-up notes make music, joined-up actions produce movement sequences, ideally with a clear and obvious beginning, middle and end.

Reflecting and making judgements – pupils describe what they and others have done; talk about what they liked in a performance; and then make practical use of this reflection to improve. Where standards in evaluating are satisfactory, there is evidence of accurate observation and awareness of the actions; understanding of differences and similarities seen in demonstrations; awareness of key features and ways to achieve them; and sensitive concern for others' feelings when discussing their work or suggesting ways that they might improve.

Year 2 Dance Programme

Pupils should be able to:

Autumn	Spring	Summer
1 Dress safely and sensibly.	1 Perform simple, basic actions such as travelling, jumping, turning and stillness, with positive, confident, correct, poised use of the body.	1 Demonstrate good body control in travelling, jumping and stillness.
2 Respond readily and quickly to instructions. Keep practising.	2 Experience and be guided in making dances with clear beginnings, middles and ends.	2 Demonstrate an enthusiasm and ability to practise to improve.
3 Improve basic actions by adding clear shapes and good poise.	3 Demonstrate increasing confidence over use of shape, space and effort.	3 Respond rhythmically to music with skill, poise, balance and co-ordination.
4 Work hard to make the lessons 'scenes of busy activity'.	4 Plan a 'Winter' dance with a partner and percussion, based on three seasonal winter words on a card.	4 Be given opportunities to explore moods and feelings through structured tasks.
5 Become body-parts aware – feet, ankles, legs, hands, arms, shoulders – and link actions in short, repeating patterns.	5 Demonstrate how good use of contrasts enhances a dance, as in winter's 'Freeze' and 'Melt'.	5 Create simple characters, expressing them through their body movements.
6 Experience working with a range of stimuli – actions, body parts, fireworks, music, poems, partner, Christmas.	6 Co-operate with a partner, often observing, commenting and, sometimes, suggesting how to improve a performance.	6 Work often with a partner to improve and extend the skills learned and to share in creating something bigger than can be achieved alone.
7 Demonstrate ability to plan and perform a series of joined-up actions, neatly.	7 Learn traditional dance steps and figures, and simple international circle dances, where class can see teacher.	7 Link movements to demonstrate an understanding of the elements of 'movement' – shape, space, effort, speed.
8 Link these movements with increasing control by using changes of direction, level, speed and tension.	8 Create simple characters and little stories in response to music. Explore feelings.	8 Make a seasonal 'Nature' dance to show how animals or plants come into being. Kittens or lambs are examples of well-known stimuli, inspiring lively action.
9 Demonstrate knowledge and understanding through actions.	9 Describe simple actions seen, using simple terms to describe.	9 Demonstrate knowledge and understanding mainly through physical actions rather than verbal expression.
10 Celebrate 'Fireworks' with good use of shape, speed, effort and direction as in rockets, Catherine wheels and bangers.		10 Learn and perform a simple, traditional British circle dance, and revise other folk dances learned previously.
11 Celebrate Christmas with 'Puppet Makers', making a simple story, expressing the weary maker, the happy puppets and the excitement of the chase.		11 Work harder for longer with greater confidence, control and versatility.
12 Describe what they and others have done and how they did it.		12 Express moods and feelings in a three-part dance about infant school days – shy start; good middle; brilliant end.
		13 Make simple, friendly judgements on how others have performed.

Year 2

Lesson Plan 1 • 30 minutes
September

Theme: *Awareness of basic actions and contrasts of shape.*

Warm-up Activities
5 minutes

Let's all join hands in a nice, big, round circle to sing and move together:

Let's join hands in one big ring, (arms swing forwards and back)
Let's join hands and let us sing, (add knees bend and stretch)
Let's join hands both high and low, (arms swing high at same time as knees stretch)
Let's drop hands and wave 'Hello!'

Let's all bounce in one big ring, (quiet, springy, upward jumps)
Let's all bounce and bounce and sing,
Let's keep bouncing, nice and slow,
Now shake hands and say 'Hello!'

Movement Skills Training
15 minutes

1 Well done, singers and dancers. That was a lively, friendly way to start. Stand in your own good space, now, and show me some of the actions that we can do on the spot to this lively, jazzy music.

2 I can see walking; marching; bouncing; skipping; stamping; running; balancing by rising and lowering on tiptoes. Practise, thinking of actions that use your feet and legs.

3 Be very clever now and add a body movement to whatever you are doing with your feet and legs. For example – stepping and clapping; bouncing and turning; stamping and gesturing. Remember, we are working on the spot – not travelling!

4 Let's look at some very good examples now.

5 Using the same lively music, let me see you travelling to visit all parts of the room. All together... best walking... best skipping... best bouncing... best hopping...

6 As you travel this time, show me different body shapes to make it more interesting. Ready... Go!... walking (tall, arms stretched upwards or feet and arms wide)... skipping (curled with arms in to sides or high, stretched leading arm and leg)... bouncing (twisted with upper body facing behind or very straight body and arms at sides)... hopping (curled, wide or stretched).

Dance — The Snake
10 minutes

1 Find a partner and stand, one behind the other, to make a little snake whose front actions will be copied by its back part. A snake's actions ripple down its body from head to tail.

2 Leaders, you are going to take your partner to different parts of the room, always looking for good spaces. Show your partner two or three actions and clear shapes to copy. Keep repeating those different actions so that you can remember them. Go!

3 Well done. Your snakes kept travelling beautifully and you are repeating your little pattern of two or three actions. Change places. The new leader can add an action on the spot before leading in to your two or three travelling actions. Begin.

4 Practice; performance; comments; improved practice.

Dance

Teaching notes and NC guidance
Development over 3 lessons

Pupils should be taught to:
a   respond readily to instructions
b   be physically active
c   be mindful of others
d   be aware of the safety risks of inappropiate clothing, footwear and jewellery.

At the start of the school year, the lesson's main emphases include:
a   establishing a tradition of immediate and whole-hearted responses to instructions. Good behaviour, expressed in listening quietly and then doing what was asked, is essential if all, including the teacher, are to enjoy action-filled, almost non-stop lessons;
b   aiming to make lessons 'scenes of busy activity', with everyone working and no-one waiting. The instant-action starting song in the circle where all can see the teacher; the lively travelling with teacher direction in the middle part of the lesson; and the simple, ongoing, partners travelling dance climax, all contribute to near non-stop action;
c   working together sensibly and co-operatively, unselfishly sharing the floor space, and expressing pleasure and appreciation for demonstrations by others;
d   all being safely and sensibly dressed.

Warm-up Activities

The teacher demonstrates two of the lines at a time, with the class watching and listening. Teacher and class repeat the sets of two lines, singing and moving, together.

Movement Skills Training

1–4 From thinking of, and practising actions on the spot, using feet and legs, pupils are challenged to add in a body movement as they were doing in the warm-up. A demonstration is essential to share the many body-and-legs dual actions that will be presented by an enthusiastic class.

5–6 From showing best travelling actions as they visit all parts of the room, pupils are now challenged to travel in a variety of ways, and include varied and interesting body shapes. The 'training', here, is in the development of an awareness of the basic travelling actions and the many contrasting body shapes that can accompany them.

The Snake Dance

1   The pairs are asked to stand about one metre apart so the follower can see the leader's feet, legs, body actions and shapes easily.

2   The teacher also emphasises that each of the two or three actions being repeated as a sequence should only last a few seconds, or for three or four travelling steps. (Unless restrained, many 'travellers' will go all around the hall, using one action only.)

3   The new leader can add a favourite action on the spot before repeating the sequence of two or three actions already created and practised.

4   Performing for others and receiving comments from others is the ideal climax to a lesson.

Year 2
Lesson Plan 2 • 30 minutes
September/October

CD TRACK 1

Theme: *Body parts awareness.*

Warm-up Activities
5 minutes

1   I will read this poem slowly. Listen carefully and show me how well you can do the actions:

Nod your head, bend your knees,
Grow as tall as Christmas trees.
On your knees, slowly fall,
Curl yourself into a ball.
Raise your head, jump up like so,
Wave your hand and say 'Hello!'

2   I will read the poem once again. Help me with the words if you remember them. Think about all the different ways our clever bodies can move.

Movement Skills Training
15 minutes

1   You danced to the poem beautifully – and remembered lots of the words. Let's see if we can practise, then remember, sets of three actions. Use your feet first. They are very important parts in movement.

2   Bounce your heels a little way off the floor, toes touching the floor. Bounce heels, bounce heels, 3, 4; bounce low, bounce low, 3, 4; springy, springy, springy, stop! Now step smartly with a lift of your front leg. Step, step, 3 and 4; stepping smartly, 3 and 4.

3   Stay where you are and stamp firmly. Stamp, stamp, 3 and 4; on the spot, 3, 4; bump, bump, bump for 4; stamp, stamp, 3 and stop!

4   Perform all three parts again, four counts to each. Ready? Bounce, bounce, heels bounce; step forwards, 3, 4; stamp, stamp, start again. Bounce, 2, 3, 4; step, 2, 3, 4; stamp, 2, 3 and stop! Good. We all kept together.

5   Hands and arms now, clapping first. Clap, 2, 3, again. Clap, 2, 3, 4. Clap, 2, 3, 4. Now let arms swing forwards and back, just like when we walk. Swings, swings, lively swings; 1, 2, 3, 4. Again, and let your shoulders twist to make the swings bigger. Swing, swing, big swings; reach, reach, 3 and 4.

6   Shake hands – as if you were shaking them to dry them. Shake, shake, shake, shake; 1, 2, 3, 4; dry them, 2, 3, 4; quick-shake, 2, 3, stop!

Dance – Clever Feet and Hands
10 minutes

1   Listen to the rhythm of the music. 1, 2, 3, 4; 1, 2, 3, 4. Keep that speed as you bounce, step, stamp for four counts. Think about and 'feel' your feet. Go! Bounce, bounce, 3, 4; step 2, 3, 4; stamp on the spot, 3, 4; bounce, 2, 3, 4; step, 2, 3, 4; stamp, 2, 3 and stop!

2   That was excellent. Three very different leg actions. Now hands only. Clap, 2, 3, 4; swing, 2, 3, 4; shake, 2, 3, 4; clap, 2, 3, 4; swing, 2, 3, 4; shake, 2, 3 and stop! Good, everyone.

3   Now, can you be very clever and join together the three leg and the three hand actions? With the music, begin. Bounce-clap, bounce-clap, bounce-clap, 4; step-swing, step-swing, step-swing, 4; stamp-shake, stamp-shake, stamp-shake, 4. (Repeat for practice.)

4   Well done. This is very difficult and you managed it splendidly. We could call our dance 'Clever Hands and Feet and Clever Girls and Boys!' Let's have half the class looking at and enjoying the other half. Then we can talk about the things we particularly liked.

Dance

Teaching notes and NC guidance
Development over 3 lessons

Pupils should be able to show control in linking actions together in ways that suit the activities.

Being able to plan and perform a series of joined-up actions neatly and with control is the main requirement within the National Curriculum. If a pupil can remember and repeat such a sequence, he or she is proving the ability to:

a   plan, showing an understanding of what was asked for
b   perform more than one skill at a time by linking actions thoughtfully
c   be able to practise and improve his or her performance.

The pattern of performing joined-up actions runs right through the lesson, as it should do right through infant school. There are eight simple actions in the warm-up, all stimulated and given a rhythm by the spoken poem.

Three sets of joined-up actions on the spot – bouncing, stepping and stamping – have a repeated rhythm, medium-speed music accompaniment in the middle of the lesson, expanded in the dance climax by adding hand and arm claps, swings and shakes. Success at this requires the total attention and whole-hearted effort sought in the previous lesson.

Warm-up Activities

1   The class can listen to two lines at a time read by the teacher. When the two lines are repeated by the teacher, the class can perform the actions.

2   Saying the words, and thinking about the many and varied actions involved and being practised, aim to develop body-parts awareness through feeling and doing.

Movement Skills Training

1–4 Pupils are praised for remembering the words in the warm-up and challenged to perform and remember the three actions – bouncing, stepping and stamping – practised in sets of three counts within a repeating pattern.

5–6 From awareness of what feet were doing, the awareness, now, is of actions the hands can perform – clapping, swinging and shaking – still within a three-part repeating pattern.

Clever Feet and Hands Dance

1   Music is introduced to give a repeating, four-count, rhythmic accompaniment to the three feet-and-leg actions sequences. Pupils are asked to 'feel' the bouncing, stepping and stamping.

2   The three-part, hands-only sequence of clapping, swinging and shaking is revised.

3   'Clever Feet and Hands' are now challenged to perform a sequence of three joined-up pairs of joined-up hands and feet actions, all in time with the rhythmic music.

4   Being able to remember, repeat, improve and present the three sets of pairs of actions is most commendable. Pupils look forward to and work hard for the demonstrations that they present, observe, comment on and learn from.

Lesson Plan 3 • 30 minutes
November

Theme: *Fireworks.*

Warm-up Activities
5 minutes

In our last lesson we created a 'Clever Feet and Hands' dance. Let's start by doing some movements that use most parts of our body. Swing the arms forwards and back, then forwards and high above your head. Bend the knees and swing the arms down to let your hands brush the floor as they swing back. Arms then swing forwards and up above the head with knees and body stretching. Again. Swing forwards, back, and forwards and up; bend down, swing arms back and forwards, and high up again. Keep practising your swinging, bending and stretching.

Movement Skills Training
15 minutes

1   What words describe a rocket's action? Whoosh? Zoom? Bang?

2   What do these actions look like? Fast, straight, streamlined?

3   Before the rocket takes off we need to light the paper fuse. It splutters and sizzles, then the long thin rocket shoots off, soaring from low to high.

4   Everyone, ready for your low, thin, streamlined start in your rocket shape. Where will you zoom to? Ready? Go!

5   How will you explode? From small to big with a scatter of your whole body? Get ready to explode, scatter and fall down. Go!

6   Let's practise again as you splutter and sizzle . . . Zoom, Whoosh . . . explode and scatter . . . twinkle, fall, glide down.

7   What are the movements of a Catherine wheel? A slow spin at the start gradually speeds up and throws out sparks. Then it slows down gradually and dies. Try the Catherine wheel movements and use your arms for spinning to stop you becoming dizzy. Show me your slow start, your speeding up, your slowing and dying.

8   What actions do the little bangers make you think of? Shooting and jumping here and there, unexpectedly in an uneven way.

9   Let me see your pattern of unexpected, quick jumping and running actions. Surprise me. Go!

10   Let's try each of the fireworks again and show me the main thing about each one. Ready, rockets? Go! Catherine wheels, go! Bangers, go! Well done. One more practice and you can accompany yourselves with your own sounds. Go!

Dance — Fireworks
10 minutes

1   That was excellent. You pleased me and surprised me. Now, you choose which one you want to be. Hands up . . . rockets . . . Catherine wheels . . . bangers. Catherine wheels go first. Go! . . . Now die away.

2   As the last Catherine wheel starts to slow... jumping bangers start now.

3   When the last two bangers only are left... Rockets sizzle, zoom, bang and scatter down like stars. Alternative ending – one rocket can stray and land in the middle of the room among all the spent fireworks lying there. The whole group can represent the unlit bonfire and start to flicker like sparks and flames, with twitching elbows and shoulders, making little fires all over. Own vocal accompaniment can be used. 'Crackle... shoot... flicker...' Slowly, the bonfire becomes quieter and dies.

Dance

Teaching notes and NC guidance
Development over 4 lessons

Pupils should be taught to develop control, co-ordination, balance, poise and elevation in the basic actions of travelling, jumping, turning, gesturing and stillness.

From the 'Clever Feet and Hands' dance of the previous lesson, we move on to clever whole bodies, working expressively to represent varied fireworks actions.

Everyone practises the three different actions in the middle of the lesson, with much questioning by the teacher to inspire a thoughtful, planned, focused response. A repeating pattern of each action is asked for so that the performers are able to remember, repeat, improve and express the movement characteristics of each one.

The dance climax, to which all the practising has led, does call for stillness while waiting one's turn; then exciting, whole-body travelling and zooming, spinning and turning, shooting and jumping; and finally gestures, as pupils shoot, explode, whirl, leap about, then crackle and flicker.

Warm-up Activities

The whole body swinging, bending and stretching can be referred to as 'our ski-swing action warm-up' and uses most joint and muscle groups, taking them to their full extension. A vocal accompaniment of 'Swish! Swish!' can be used with the long arm swings.

Movement Skills Training

In contrast to the direct teaching of the previous lesson where the pupils were given the exact nature of the bounces, steps and stamps by the teacher (e.g. 'bounce low, springy'; 'step smartly with lift of front foot', etc.), the teacher is now continually challenging and questioning the class to make them think about and plan their own responses, asking: 'What kind of actions?' (rockets, Catherine wheel, little bangers),'Where will you zoom to?' and challenging 'Show me...'; 'Let me see...'.

In this shared-choice teaching style the teacher decides the nature of the activity and the class decide the actual actions. Shared choice leads to a wide variety of results and an expanded class and teacher repertoire. The wide use of imagery and imagination helps the class to express themselves more clearly. 'Zooming' when imagining that you are moving like a rocket makes the action much easier to express than if you are simply trying to zoom as a way of travelling.

Fireworks Dance

The dance performance climax of the lesson is a good example of a shared-choice presentation. Pupils decide which firework they will represent and the teacher decides the order of the dance itself – Catherine wheel start; jumping bangers middle; and rockets ending. The teacher is the main observer of the whole dance, but each of the three groups can watch the other two while waiting their turn to start, or after performing.

Lesson Plan 4 • 30 minutes
December

Theme: *Christmas and toys.*

Warm-up Activities
5 minutes

1 Find a partner for 'Follow My Leader'. The leader pretends the partner is just learning to move and has to be shown, very carefully, how to use the different parts of the body. Make your movements 'larger than life' and let's see if you can make a little pattern of three actions, exactly together.

2 Following partner, you lead now and show me your 'larger than life' ways to move feet, legs, arms, shoulders, or the whole body.

Movement Skills Training
15 minutes

1 Keep the same partner, well spaced out all over the room, facing each other. One of you will be the puppet maker with your hammer and chisel. The other will be the still, solid block of wood.

2 Puppet maker, chisel out the head shape. Show your puppet how a head can move up, down, side to side, and rotate. Puppet, copy.

3 Puppet maker, work on the shoulders and show how they can lift and lower, go forwards and back, and do circular motions.

4 Arms are shaped next with long, up-and-down chisel movements. The bending, stretching, swinging and circling are then copied.

5 The body shape and the big body movements of bending, stretching, twisting and turning are made and demonstrated.

6 Legs are the most important body part. The puppet maker has to crouch low to shape out the legs and feet. Big actions of bending to the front and sides and swinging are shown and copied on the spot.

7 Legs can do much more than swing, bend and step on the spot. They can take you to all parts of the room. Some puppet makers choose to do 'Follow My Leader' with their puppets. Others, with hands high above the puppet's head, suspend them from strings. Mirroring or dangling, the puppets are guided through the varied travelling actions. They walk, skip, run, hop, bounce, jump with full use of the neck, arms, shoulders and legs just created.

Dance — Puppet Makers
10 minutes

Music: Beethoven's 9th, Choral Symphony – *Ode to Joy*

1 From the beginning with the still, solid lump of wood, the puppet makers hammer and chisel the shape of head, shoulders, arms, body, feet and legs. At each stage, they demonstrate and lead the growing puppet through the body movements of each. Puppet makers travel with their own puppets as they visit all parts of the room. Movements are 'larger than life'.

2 All this hammering, chiselling and moving has been hard work. The puppets are hung up on a hook in the workshop and the puppet makers lie down for a well-earned rest and sleep on the floor.

3 The puppets have enjoyed their play-like travels so much that they jump down off their wall hooks and all dance round.

4 The puppet makers waken and are angry to see their puppets out of place. They chase after their own puppet who dodges away.

5 Puppets are caught and gripped firmly with one hand. The other hand points and gestures 'Naughty puppet! Behave yourself!'

Dance

Teaching notes and NC guidance
Development over 4 lessons

Pupils should be taught to explore feelings and develop their response to music through Dance by using rhythmic responses. Pupils should be able to improve performance, through practice, alone and with a partner.

In this easy dance the pupils can almost be talked through the whole dance by the teacher, who guides them through the timings of each part. 'Chisel out the head shape, front, sides, back, top. Now show your puppet how its head can move. Puppets, watch and copy.' A repeating pattern at each stage will be helpful in remembering, repeating and improving the dance. 'Show your puppet how legs can swing forwards and back, forwards and back; step, step on the spot; swing to one side, swing to other side; swing forwards and back, forwards and back; step, step, on the spot; swing to one side, swing to other side.'

   'Feelings' being expressed will include the weariness of the hard-working puppet makers as they sag slowly to rest on the floor; the happiness of the puppets as they travel and try out all the enjoyable play-like movements possible in their clever bodies; the surprise and annoyance of the puppet makers when they waken and see the badly behaved puppets at the games of chase.

Warm-up Activities

Partners face each other, a metre apart, and perform large movements of body parts slowly, allowing partners to keep exactly together. A varied, repeating, linked trio of activities might include one for legs; one for arms; and one for the whole body.

Movement Skills Training

The teacher, with a partner, but without any music, demonstrates briefly the pattern of chiselling each part, and then showing the growing puppet how that part can move. 'No touching any part of your partner as you make head, shoulders, arms, body or legs' must be emphasised or pupils will make contact with their imaginary hammers and chisels.

Puppet Makers Dance

1   With the music now, and with the teacher's continuous reminder of the body parts to be demonstrated by the puppet maker and practised by the emerging puppet, the complete puppet is built out of the starting block of wood. 'Hold your puppet on a string, walking behind the puppet' is the reminder as the finished puppet is allowed to travel, using all the body parts to try them out while moving. We want these movements to be 'larger than life' once again.

2–3 Hard-working, tired puppet makers hang their puppets on a hook and lie down for their well-earned rest. Like young children, the puppets jump from their hooks and dance all around the room.

4–5 Puppet makers, disturbed by the sound of puppets dashing around, jump up and chase after their own puppet. When the music stops, the puppet makers catch and hold their puppet.

Lesson Plan 5 • 30 minutes
January

Theme: *Winter.*

Warm-up Activities
5 minutes

Let's sing and move to keep warm, pretending we are outside:

This is the way we skip to keep warm,
skip to keep warm, skip to keep warm,
This is the way we skip to keep warm,
on a cold and frosty morning

This is the way we big bend and stretch,
big bend and stretch, big bend and stretch,
    (bend knees to touch floor, high stretch)
This is the way we big bend and stretch,
on a cold and frosty morning.

(Repeat several times.)

Movement Skills Training
15 minutes

1 If I asked you to do a 'Winter' drawing, what would you do?

2 'Snowflakes falling' is a good answer, thank you. Can you all move like a snowflake, slowly, gently, turning, hovering, falling?

3 'Wind bending the trees' is another good answer, thank you. Show me how the wind's strong, big, rushing movement is different from the snowflake's.

4 'Ice in a stream' is another excellent answer, thank you. Let me see you flowing like a stream. When I call 'Freeze!' show me how quickly you can stiffen into your rigid, jagged, icy shape.

Dance — Winter
10 minutes

WIND: SWOOSH, WHIRL, DROP
SNOWFLAKE: FLOAT, HOVER, SINK
STREAM: RUSH, FREEZE, MELT

1 Find a partner. One of you will collect a card and the other will pick up a piece of percussion.

2 Find a good floor space and look at the three action words on your card. Please do not look at other couples' cards. Three different cards are being used for our 'Winter' dance. Each card also tells you what is doing the three actions.

3 Dancing partner, perform your three actions carefully for your partner to watch and then make helpful comments. Start when ready – without any percussion sounds at this stage.

4 Well done. Dancers, sit down and be given some friendly, helpful advice to improve your performance. Were the actions clear? Were the body shapes full and clear? Was the speed right?

5 The same dancer again, please. Partner with percussion, you may quietly accompany your partner, starting and stopping to make the three actions separate. Begin when ready, please.

6 Well done, everyone. The improvements were obvious. Now change places. No accompaniment this time. New dancer, begin when ready.

7 Dancers, sit down and listen to the helpful comments.

8 Same dancers practise again, using the good advice received.

Dance

Teaching notes and NC guidance
Development over 4 lessons

Pupils should be involved in the continuous process of planning, performing and evaluating.

As well as asking him or herself, 'Was my lesson filled with worthwhile, enjoyable and challenging activity, flowing almost non-stop from start to finish?' the teacher also needs to check, 'Did I provide opportunities for thoughtful planning, challenging the pupils to think ahead to try to see an intended outcome? Did the lesson build up to an end-of-lesson performance of a created dance? Somewhere in the lesson did I provide opportunities for the class to see a demonstration and make friendly, helpful comments, evaluating what they had seen?'

In the shared-choice teaching method used in the lesson, the teacher, with the help of action words on cards, decides the nature of the activity. The pupils then plan and decide the precise actions to be practised, repeated, improved and eventually presented. The observing partner has to watch carefully to identify the main feature of the actions, reflect on their accuracy, and then sensitively suggest ways to bring about an improvement.

Warm-up Activities

With an instant start, the teacher sings out the words of this well-known poem and starts to perform the actions which the class will immediately start to copy. Other ideas for keeping warm in winter might include *'This is the way we dance in the hall, dance in the hall'* and *'This is the way we chase outside, chase outside.'*

Movement Skills Training

From moving bodies trying to keep warm in winter, we move on to imagery and trying to express wintry features suggested by the class, imagining how they might move. Such use of imagination makes the actions 'like snowflakes, trees in the wind, ice in a stream' much easier to understand, plan and represent. The teacher's 'Show me...; Can you...?; Let me see...' challenges the class to produce focused, thoughtful, varied, good-quality movements.

Winter Dance

1–3 One partner sits with the card on the floor in front of him or her. The dancing partner stands beside the inactive one, ready to dance onto the small 'stage' in front of them. The dancing partner performs each of the three actions for a time limit set by the teacher. 'First action to bring you on to your little stage... go! Second action... begin! Final action... now!'

4–5 Dancers sit down beside the observing partners to be given encouragement for good points, and help to make the dance better by suggested improvements. Same dancer, after receiving advice, repeats the three actions, accompanied this time by the percussion played by the partner. The responsibility for the timing is given to the partner with the percussion.

6–8 Partners change over and the new dancer, after their experience as teacher-coach, should be able to present a good performance with neat actions, clear shapes, and good use of space and effort. Once again, the new dancers sit to be advised and helped by the observing partner, who is asked to 'Tell your partner something that you particularly liked and tell them one thing that might improve the performance' to help them as they perform again.

Lesson Plan 6 • 30 minutes
February

Theme: *Traditional dance.*

Warm-up Activities
5 minutes

1 Partners, travel side by side, keeping in time with the music. One of you will decide your actions, which each take eight bars of the music. Try to include two or three different actions. A change of direction on '8' looks very attractive.

2 Other partner, can you decide on actions to take your pair apart and then bring you together again? Separate for eight counts, then come together again for eight counts.

3 Partners, practise a four-part repeating pattern of travelling side by side; parting; closing; travelling together.

Teach a Dance — Djatchko Kolo (Yugoslavian Folk Dance)
20 minutes

Music: *Djatchko Kolo*, Society for International Folk Dancing (cassette and book 3)

Formation: An open circle with teacher at right hand open end. This simple dance can be learned easily, with the teacher calling out and demonstrating each movement straight away with the music, and the class copying the teacher.

Figure A

Bar 1	Beat 1	Step right foot to right.
	2	Close left foot to right foot.
	3	Step right foot to right.
	4	Swing left foot across right foot.
Bar 2	Beats 1–4	Repeat Bar 1 to the left, starting with left foot.
Bars 3 & 4		Repeat all of above.

Figure B

Bar 5	Beat 1	Step right foot to right.
	2	Swing left foot across right foot.
	3	Step left foot to left.
	4	Swing right foot across left foot.
Bar 6	Beats 1–4	Repeat Bar 5.

Figure C

| Bars 7 & 8 | Starting with right foot, perform seven little walking steps to right and point heel of left foot on the floor on '8'. |
| Bars 9 & 10 | Seven steps to left and point heel of right foot on the floor on '8'. |

Keep repeating dance from beginning.

Revise a Favourite Dance
5 minutes

Ideally, this favourite dance, often chosen by the pupils, will contrast with the new dance of this lesson. It could be a revision of January's 'Winter' Dance.

Dance

Teaching notes and NC guidance
Development over 4 lessons

Pupils should be taught to perform movements or patterns, including some from existing dance traditions. Pupils should be able to show control in linking actions together.

A traditional Dance lesson has many attractions. The warm-up gives the lesson a lively, repeating, rhythmic start, always with the possibility of development into enjoyable partner activity. The four-part repeating pattern gives the opportunity for varied, creative activity, which is a good balance to the formal steps and figures of the folk dance.

When the steps and patterns of the dance are easy, as here, pupils quickly gain the pleasure of learning, mastering, repeating and improving another dance to add to their expanding repertoire. The circle formation lends itself to all pupils being able to see and copy the teacher's lead from start to finish. The slow rhythm at the start of the dance, accompanied by the teacher's rhythmic accompaniment of the simple actions, provides an almost instantly learned dance. Improvement comes with repetitions of the dance, with a different emphasis each time. 'Keep the circle round; grip with hands higher than elbows; erect posture throughout; neat steps and swings.'

Warm-up Activities

1   An instant start with number one partner showing the two or three simple actions being repeated in time with the eight-count pattern of the music. The suggested change of direction will be helpful anyway as partners approach a wall or other couples.

2   Number two partner is challenged to plan actions suitable for parting and closing, taking eight counts for each. Cross-over steps and a step-close chasse are neat and do not take up too much space.

3   'Showing control in linking actions' is the challenge. 'Can you show me your joined-up, four-part sequence of joined-up travelling actions; joined-up parting and closing actions; and joined-up travelling together?'

Teach a Dance – Djatchko Kolo (Yugoslavian Folk Dance)

The combination of very slow music, simple steps and a teacher in the circle demonstrating each figure makes this an easy dance to teach. The teacher's accompanying commentary for the first figure 'Step right, close left, step right, swing left; step left, close right, step left, swing right' is easy to understand and follow and is helped by the whole circle and the teacher moving in the correct directions.

Figures 2 and 3 are equally simple to learn and follow; repetition helps to reinforce the learning.

Revise a Favourite Dance

Ease of learning and a successful double performance of the lesson's dance usually leaves enough time for a competent, enthusiastic class to be told, 'Well done. You worked really well and did that new dance brilliantly. Would anyone like to suggest a different dance for us to finish with? A more lively dance, not in a circle, and one that you yourselves created might be a good contrast.'

Lesson Plan 7 • 30 minutes
March

Theme: *Creating simple characters in response to music.*

Warm-up Activities
5 minutes

1. Let's warm up with some actions that might describe different types of people. Off we go, proud soldiers. March, march, swing your arms; left, right, left, right; lift your knees, lift your arms; 1, 2, 3, 4.

2. Well done, proud soldiers. Ready again? Dithery person, here and there; ooops, I don't know where I'm going; side to side, forwards and back; turn around, change my mind.

3. Well dithered! One more. Ready? Tired person, flop about; dangling arms and heavy head; dragging legs and sagging knees.

Movement Skills Training
15 minutes

1. Listen to the slow, swaggering rhythm of the music. Feel the 1, 2, 3, 4 repeating beat and imagine yourself as someone very important, stepping out confidently to it.

2. Let's try some proud, slow steps, just like a very self-confident policeman or policewoman might do. Go!

3. Well done. This time, pretend you are on your beat, patrolling the streets where you live. Turn corners; cross roads, looking right, left, right; and let your cocky head and shoulders say 'All's well. We don't have any baddies around here.'

4. That was excellent. You all look very cocky and proud. Now let's try some suspicious 'Baddie' movements as if you are sneaking along behind one of these very special coppers, silently keeping just out of sight. Use little runs, dodging behind bushes, letter boxes, in driveways or in doorways. Off you go!

5. Sometimes you will be close behind, copying the swaggering, cocky walking – and being a little bit cocky yourself. You can stop and start together; sometimes freeze while the copper looks around; even pretend to be simply reading a paper or looking at your watch. Let's pretend to be self-confident baddies. Go!

Dance — Cops and Robbers
10 minutes

Music: The 'Pink Panther' theme from *The Pink Panther* **by Henry Mancini and his Orchestra**

1. Find a partner and decide who is the copper and who is the robber. Stand ready for our practice, our little game of chase. Let's see if the cops can do a repeating pattern of travelling so that the baddie can also repeat his or her pattern of secret following, weaving in and out, behind, side to side, close-up copying and freezing still. Start with the music.

2. Well done, cocky cops and robbers. This time I will stop the music as a signal for the copper to turn suddenly and catch the baddie. Running away is not allowed, you baddies! The goodies will grab hold with one hand and hold their truncheons above their partner's head with the other hand, expressing 'Gotcha!' The poor loser will express 'It's a fair cop, officer'. Ready? Go! (Let pupils perform for about one minute, then the music is suddenly stopped.)

3. Hold your positions, please. Well done. Now relax and we'll look at each half of the class in turn to see the many brilliant ideas you have created. You can tell me which ones you like.

Dance

Teaching notes and NC guidance
Development over 4 lessons

Pupils should be taught to express and communicate moods, ideas and feelings, and develop their responses to music.

The 'feelings' referred to include the interesting contrast in the movement expressions of the confident, self-assured, slightly arrogant, swaggering policeman or policewoman, and the movement expressions of the equally cocky, self-assured, sometimes cheeky robber.

Pupils practise each of the two parts separately, sometimes adding individual, funny mannerisms to their big swaggering walkabout. A standing cop shines the toes on the back of the other trouser leg; sticks thumbs through the braces; twirls the baton; waves to the adoring public; occasionally looks bored at such a crime-free existence.

The pursuing robber, bursting with self-assurance, zigzags along, out of sight and out of hearing of the copper, sometimes hiding, then rushing after him or her. Occasionally, the cockiness leads to a close shadowing, mimicking the copper's every move. Both use larger than life, big body movements to express how pleased they are with themselves.

Warm-up Activities

The use of imagery, with pupils pretending and imagining that they are moving like certain kinds of people, makes it easier to express pride, ditheriness or tiredness. Trying to express such feelings, in isolation, without reference to persons of those types, is much harder.

Movement Skills Training

1   The music invites a shoulder-swaggering, high-stepping, arm-swinging walk, 'expressing moods and feelings' as the class imagines that they are brilliant, or are suddenly transformed into some VIP, arrogantly looking from side to side, to check that all are admiring them.

2–3 Along with their proud, slow steps, the coppers are asked to try to plan and add some other copper-like actions of their own. These gestures all need to be shared and admired. The bored yawns and the looks at the wristwatch all infer 'There's no baddies around here. We've cleaned up the area.'

4–5 Pupils are challenged to plan where the baddies will go, keeping out of sight, as they pursue their copper. 'Expressing ideas' includes ways to look innocent when the copper turns around.

Cops and Robbers Dance

Couples are given the difficult challenge of planning and repeating the pathways followed in travelling and pursuing. A pattern of three or four proud, cop-like actions along a repeating route with the robber's repeated pattern of zigzagging from tree to doorway; dropping down low out of sight; close behind mimicking; and a quick-thinking innocent gesture, for example, will give observers plenty to 'look out for and tell me what you liked' during the demonstrations later. The music is stopped as the signal for the copper to apprehend the robber. Each then expresses the appropriate feelings after victory and defeat.

Lesson Plan 8 • 30 minutes
April

Theme: *Clowns.*

Warm-up Activities
5 minutes

1 Let's try a warm-up that I call '8:4:2' and see if you can keep up with me. Eight skips forwards... go! Skip, 2, 3, 4, 5, 6, 7, stop!

2 Good. You all started and stopped with me. Now an easy four steps backwards... go! Step, 2, 3 and stop!

3 We've gone forwards. We've gone backwards. What direction do you think we will go next? Yes, sideways with two chasse steps. Do it slowly with me. Step to the side; close feet together; step to the side; close feet together. Now do it a little bit quicker. Side step, close; side step, close. Well done. Now let's try the whole of our '8:4:2'. Skip forwards, 3, 4, 5, 6, 7, 8; step backwards, 3, 4; side step, close, side step, close. Excellent. Again... go!

Movement Skills Training
15 minutes

1 In our last lesson we thought about and moved like several different sorts of people – soldiers, ditherers, tired people and cops and robbers. At Easter time, as at Christmas time, there are often circuses to visit. What do you call the funny performers in a circus? Yes, clowns.

2 Show me a funny clown walk, please. Can you turn your toes in a long way, swing your arms across your chest, and swing your shoulders up and down a long way?

3 You might try your funny walk going backwards and sideways as well as forwards. Four steps each way would be a nice pattern.

4 Try a funny walk on your heels, or your toes, or one of each. Add lots of funny, big, swinging arm, shoulder and head movements.

5 Clowns do lots of balancing on one foot and then suddenly stumble, nearly falling down as they do little running steps to save themselves. Show me your funny balance shapes and your wobbling, stumbling quick steps to balance still again.

6 Sometimes they do lose balance and sit down on their bottom. Show me a balance on your bottom with legs stuck up in the air.

7 Now twist over on to your tummy and show me another funny balance, with arms and legs lifted and doing swimming actions.

Dance — The Clowns
10 minutes

Music: TV Sport from *Festival of Music* by Central Band of the R.A.F.

1 Practise a pattern of funny walks, funny balances, staggers and runs to save yourself, and funny stumbles into a balance on your bottom or chest, or one of each. Then jump up like 'Jack In The Box'.

2 Find a partner and pretend your partner needs cheering up. Find a good space for your little circus ring. One of you sit down as a spectator. The other one does his or her clown dance to include some funny walking, funny balancing, wobbling, staggering, and then a sit down and funny balance on your bottom or front, or both.

3 Well done. Have one more practice. You can use our 8:4:2 pattern if you like – eight funny walks, four funny balances, wobbles and staggering about, and two balances, one on seat and one on chest.

4 Hands up all the spectators who laughed because you were amused? Can anyone tell me what you thought was good fun?

5 Change over now to a new clown and a new spectator. Start when you are ready. Clowns, dancers, give us a good laugh, please.

Dance

Teaching notes and NC guidance
Development over 4 lessons

Pupils should be able to show that they can improve performance, through practice, alone and with a partner.

From performing the movement characteristics of hyper-confident cops and robbers, we move on to show the equally exaggerated typical movements of a circus clown. The eventual performance by the clown has far greater potential for variety and interest, and for a repeating pattern of funny movements. The funny walking in all directions on all parts of the feet, the unstable, wobbly balancing on feet, the staggering run to regain balance, and the falling to balance on seat or back can all be fitted into a repeating, contrasting pattern that aids remembering and improvement.

Partners' observations and comments also aid the altering, adapting and extending that promote further planning and an improved performance.

Warm-up Activities

This individual, three-part, repeating and reducing sequence will keep pupils concentrating to remember: (a) the three different actions – skips, steps and chasse steps; (b) the three different directions – forwards, backwards and sideways; and (c) the three different lengths of the phrases – eight skips, four steps and two chasse steps.

Movement Skills Training

After the experience gained in expressing, through body movements, the personality, feelings and moods of cops and robbers in the previous lesson, moving as a clown and expressing the feelings and personalities of clowns should be easier to achieve in this lesson. After the 'Show me a funny clown walk, please,' the teacher is at his or her busiest in the middle part of the lesson, questioning, challenging, encouraging, as well as giving direct advice and suggestions for improvement. Good demonstrations showing ideal outcomes and responses will be a regular feature within the 'training' part of the lesson. Pupils remember what they see and the important elements within movement – shapes, directions, effort – will be more clearly understood through demonstrations than through explanations alone.

Clown Dance

1   The many separate features of clown-like actions – funny walks and balances, staggers, stumbles and balances on bottom or chest – all practised, repeated and improved in the middle of the lesson, are here linked into a four-part sequence.

2–5 Performing for your own partner in the typical performer and spectator setting of a small circus ring is a different, new and challenging experience for partners, requiring larger-than-life actions to make them realistic. Clowns need to perform strongly to be seen by spectators in the very back of the rows of seats. The 8:4:2 pattern of the start of the lesson is a good guide for a satisfactory length of performance in the created dance climax of the end of the lesson.

Lesson Plan 9 • 30 minutes
May

Theme: *Kittens.*

Warm-up Activities
5 minutes

1   Lots of baby animals are born in spring and they have to learn how to use their muscles to move.

2   With silent feet, weave in and out of one another, trying out the different ways your legs can travel. If you were a baby animal – lamb, puppy, kitten – you might try a little run and jump up.

3   Run a little way, jump high, then bend down towards the ground for a silent landing. Jump up and do a bendy, squashy landing. A baby animal doesn't want to hurt its bones and lands gently.

4   Often the baby animal springs up, twists in the air, and lands facing another way. Try a jump, twist and gentle landing.

Movement Skills Training
15 minutes

1   Let's think about how a kitten might try out its muscles. Lie curled up small on the carpet in your home. Can you roll over from one side of your body to the other side? Roll and roll; a curled-up roll; side to side; roll and roll. Well done, kittens.

2   Now sit up tall, and stretch out your body. Stretch up one paw, 1–4; pull it down, 5–8; stretch up the other paw, 1–4; pull it down, 5–8; stretch up both paws at the same time and this time try out your claws, 1–4; pull in your claws and paws, 5–8.

3   On hands and knees, try a whole-body stretch and arch up high, 1–4; relax down again, 5–8; whole body arch high, 1–4; relax down again, 5–8.

4   Jump up from your carpet. Go out into your garden and try a run and a jump, landing gently. Not a sound! Do it two or three times and you can try a clever twist to land facing a different way.

5   Here's a high fence. Run and jump high to balance and walk along it, forwards then backwards, forwards then backwards.

6   Be clever and balance on one foot only on the fence, stretching out all parts of your body. Balance again, on the other foot.

7   It's time to go indoors. Jump down from your high fence and do a soft, squashy landing. Go back to your carpet starting places.

Dance – Kittens
10 minutes

1   All lie curled up small on your nice soft carpet. Roll over from one side of your body to the other side. Roll and roll.

2   Sit up tall and straight and try out one paw as you stretch, 2, 3, 4; pull in, 2, 3, 4; other paw, stretch, 2, 3, 4; pull in, 2, 3, 4; both paws and claws, stretch, 2, 3, 4; pull in, 2, 3, 4.

3   On your hands and knees, try out your whole body arching up... and down... and arch high up... and relax down.

4   Jump up and go out into the garden for a run and jump and a soft landing. Run, jump, land. Run, jump and twist and land. Now a really high jump up on to the fence.

5   Balance-walk slowly forwards, backwards, forwards, backwards. Now on one foot only, stretch everything. On to the other foot and a big stretch of your whole body. Really stretch.

6   Jump down very gently and walk back to your nice soft carpet.

7   Repetition; performance; comments; improved practice.

Dance

Teaching notes and NC guidance
Development over 4 lessons

Pupils should be taught to adopt the best possible posture and use of the body as they perform imaginatively. Pupils should be able to show control in linking actions together.

The body's posture and use are more evident during whole-body movements such as bending, stretching, twisting, turning and arching than when we do the everyday actions of travelling using our legs. These whole-body movements are also performed slowly, which means that they can be performed thoughtfully and to the limits of the joints concerned.

In the 'Kittens' dance, movements are used to express the typical movement characteristics of a young animal recently born in Spring. Pupils are asked to be conscious of their posture and to be aware of the repeating patterns of joined-up movements as an aid to remembering, repeating and improving the dance with all its contrasts of action and use of space.

Warm-up Activities

1–2 Throughout the lesson, imagery helps our aim of learning and imagining how young baby animals learn to use their muscles to move, soon after their birth in Spring. The little run and jump and the uncertain, hither-and-thither travelling, are typical of young kittens and lambs.

3–4 The soft and careful use of feet and legs in running is repeated in the jumps and squashy landings, protecting young bones and joints. A teacher demonstration, starting facing one end of the hall, then running and jumping to turn in the air, landing to face the other end of the hall, is a popular challenge.

Movement Skills Training

1 The 'Let's think about how a kitten might try out its muscles' start to the training part of the lesson puts the class 'in the picture' straight away and focuses their attention on the movements concerned. A teacher demonstration of the side-to-side rolls will show the hands clasped under the bent knees to make the whole spine rounded from shoulders to seat.

2 Sitting tall after being curled, pupils slowly stretch and feel the paws reaching up and down, followed by the dual action of paws and claws.

3 The strong arch high on hands and feet alternates with the whole body lowering without touching the floor. This is a strong exercise, arching or bridging, on hands and feet only.

4–6 The run and jump in the garden can include the jump and turn with a squashy landing of the warm-up. The run and jump high on to the garden fence is followed by a slow, careful balance-walk forwards and backwards, with four steps each way, then repeated. At the end of each forwards and back travel, pupils are asked, 'Can you be a clever kitten and stand on one paw only on your fence?' The class, like the teacher, will discover that they have one leg that is better and more reliable for balancing on.

7 The jump down from the fence needs to be done softly and with a nice, squashy landing on to the young feet and legs of our kittens, before they return to their own starting places.

Kittens Dance

After the stage-by-stage teaching of the middle part of the lesson, pupils now dance the whole dance, guided and reminded by the teacher's demonstrations and commentary.

Lesson Plan 10 • 30 minutes
June

CD TRACKS 7 + 12

Theme: *Traditional dance.*

Warm-up Activities
5 minutes

1   Join hands with your partner in a big circle. Stand, side by side, all facing anti-clockwise.

2   Travel around in the circle with eight skipping steps.

3   Face your partner, without touching, and do four setting steps. (Step to right, close left to right, step on right; Step to left, close right to left, step on left.) 1... 2, 3; 2... 2, 3; right... 2, 3; left... 2, 3.

4   Change places with your partner, holding hands for four counts.

5   Face your partner again and do four setting steps on the spot.

6   Change places with your partner, holding hands for four counts.

7   Perform eight skipping steps forwards, dancing side by side, hands joined.

8   Keep repeating this 32-count (4 × 8-count) pattern.

Teach a Dance — Pat-A-Cake Polka (English Folk Dance)
20 minutes

Music: *Pat-A-Cake Polka* by Blue Mountain Band

Formation: A double circle with boys' backs to the centre. Directions given are those of the dancer on the inside of the circle.

Figure A: Boys, hold both of your partner's hands, facing sideways. Moving anti-clockwise, dance 'heel and toe' and two chasse steps (illustrated) to the boys' left. (Touch floor with leading heel, then toes, then the quick chasse action, left, right, left), and repeat back again to boys' right (leading heel and toe each time). Repeat the whole movement,

using a good spring at the start of each movement. 'Heel, toe, chasse, 2, 3; heel, toe, 1, 2, 3.'

Figure B: Partners clap right hands together three times. Partners clap left hands together three times. Partners clap both hands together three times. Partners clap own knees three times.

Figure C: Boy turns partner around for four counts to the starting position to repeat the dance, or does a quick two-count turn followed by boy moving on one place, anti-clockwise, to make the dance progressive, dancing next with a new partner.

Repeat.

Revise a Favourite Dance
5 minutes

To provide the variety and contrast which is always an attractive feature of a Dance lesson, it is recommended that this dance is not danced in a circle formation. Ideally, also, it will be one of a more modern, creative, less traditional type.

Dance

Teaching notes and NC guidance
Development over 4 lessons

Pupils should be taught to perform movements or patterns, including some from existing dance traditions and different times and cultures. Pupils should be able to show control in linking actions together in ways that suit the activities.

The dance has an A:B:C repeating pattern of movement actions that are linked together. 'A' is the chasse left and right, twice, 'B' is the quick hand-clapping and 'C' is the turning with your partner, back to your own place, ready to start again. The NC required patterns of movement and the linking of actions together are both well represented in this, as in all traditional dances.

Because of the high speed of this dance, it is essential that the teacher vocally accompanies the actions, phrase by phrase, as a reminder to the pupils, especially focussing on their high speed. 'Heel, toe, side, 2, 3; heel, toe, side, 2, 3; heel, toe, chasse left; heel, toe, chasse right' and (clapping) 'Right, 2, 3; left, 2, 3; both, 2, 3; knees', both of which will be helped further by the teacher joining in with the actions.

Warm-up Activities

1   In a side-by-side, hands-held position, hands should be held above bent-elbows height.

2   In the anti-clockwise skipping, pupils are asked to 'Keep your nice big circle shape.'

3-6 Setting on the spot and changing places, hands held, then setting again on the spot and changing places again, hands held, is quite difficult. If pupils have not been taught the setting step, a quick right, left, right; left, right, left stepping on the spot will suffice. In turning, hands are again held above bent-elbow height, with the pupil whose hands are underneath doing the guiding.

7   The dance ends as it started with eight anti-clockwise travelling steps with partners' hands joined.

Teach a Dance – Pat-A-Cake-Polka (English Folk Dance)

Figure A: In the double circle of couples with hands joined, the pupils with their backs to the centre are told that they are dancing the boys' part – even if pairs of boys and pairs of girls are in the habit of dancing together. The teacher explains that he or she is speaking to the pupil dancing the boys' part because a direction applying to that dancer is involved. The 'Heel, toe, chasse left; heel toe, chasse right', taught slowly without any music at this stage, will, of course, be the opposite direction for the ones in the outer circle. The pupil dancing the boy's part, with back to centre, guides his or her partner in the right direction with hands held above bent-elbow height, and with guiding partner's hands underneath, taking the weight. Movement is repeated.

Figure B: Still without music while learning the dance, the teacher and a partner demonstrate the rapid clapping of 'Right, 2, 3; left, 2, 3; both, 2, 3; own knees, 2, 3.' All practise to the teacher's commentary reminder.

Figure C: The four-count turn, using two hands to help each other, is slow and easy, and the teacher needs to emphasise that there is plenty of time to complete the turn.

Dance is repeated, with music, accompanied by the teacher's continuous reminder/commentary.

Year 2

Lesson Plan 11 • 30 minutes
July

CD TRACK 3

Theme: *Friendships.*

Warm-up Activities
5 minutes

1 Let's remind ourselves of the friendly way we joined hands and sang when you started school:

   Let's join hands in one big ring,
   Let's join hands and let us sing,
   Let's join hands, both high and low,
   Let's drop hands and wave 'Hello!'

2 Now let's skip to this jazzy music for eight counts, change direction and go off again. Skip, 2, 3, 4, 5, 6, change direction; skip, 2, 3, 4, 5, 6, change again; skip, 2, 3, 4, 5, 6, 7, stop!

3 Now, meet and give a friendly touch to someone coming towards you, saying 'Hello! Hello!' Ready? Skip, 2, 3, 4, 5, 6, change direction; skip, 2, 3, 4, 5, meet and 'Hello! Hello!' – keep going!

Movement Skills Training
10 minutes

1 Think about the time you started school, not knowing anyone in your class. Show me how you might have walked, skipped or run around the playground, all by yourself.

2 Walk in and out of one another, looking at those coming towards you. Show me a friendly smile, wave or nod your head as you pass them.

3 When I beat the drum, make a friendly contact with the nearest person: a handshake; friendly touch on the shoulder; flat hand to hand.

4 As you grew older you became good at playing with others. Find a partner, sit down and decide on a shared activity you enjoy. Dance together; throw and catch; walk.

Dance — Friendships
15 minutes

1 Well done. Lots of good fun ideas. Can you now agree a three- or four-part pattern to make your sequence more interesting. Each of you suggest one or two ideas for your shared, repeating activity. Practise when you are ready.

2 Well done. Your repeating patterns improve each time. Remember them for later. Now go and stand by yourself for the start of our 'Friendships' dance, pretending it is your first day at school.

3 Playing all by yourselves, ready, begin! Find good spaces, well away from others. Be lively, please!

4 Change to walking in and out of others, looking at, smiling, waving or nodding your head.

5 On my drum beat, stop and make a friendly, gentle contact with the nearest person, then move on.

6 When my drum sounds twice, go to your partner and start your shared, enjoyable activity. Try to repeat and improve it.

7 Very well done. Let's look at each half of the class in turn, demonstrating the last part of the dance. Tell me what you liked.

8 Thank you for your excellent performances and your friendly, helpful comments. Now, let's all join hands in a big, friendly circle and sing:

   Let's join hands, getting all together,
   Let's join hands in a circle round,
   In we skip, good friends together,
   Clap our hands and turn around.
   Hands joined again, keeping close together,
   Skipping back out, off we go,
   Our joined-up hands swing high and low,
   Now we shake hands and say 'Hello!'

Dance

Teaching notes and NC guidance
Development over 4 lessons

Pupils should be able to show that they are able to involve themselves in the continuous process of planning, performing and evaluating.

Ideally, they will be working harder for longer in almost non-stop action, displaying greater control and versatility. There should be an impression of confidence, enthusiasm and enjoyment as they stamp the work with their own personality.

Warm-up Activities

1   The sociable 'togetherness' potential of good Physical Education lessons was evident in the 'Let's join hands and wave "Hello!"' of the very first lesson of the Reception Year programme. Since then, in Dance lessons, pupils will have joined hands in a friendly way hundreds of times.

2–3   After skipping for six counts and changing direction on counts 7 and 8, pupils now alternate skipping for six with a direction change on counts 7 and 8 and skipping for six and giving a friendly hand touch to someone on counts 7 and 8, with a 'Hello! Hello!'

Movement Skills Training

1   In these four stages of infant-school social development, pupils start as shy individuals, walking, skipping, running or galloping alone at play time in the playground. No-one is making any form of communication with anyone else.

2   As a start to socialising, pupils now look at and make friendly, smiling gestures and waves as they pass others near to them. A nod of the head in someone's direction is always pleasant to give and to receive.

3   'When I sound the drum, can you stop and show me how you can make a friendly contact with the nearest person? Please try to surprise me with interesting and maybe unusual body parts making contact – always in a gentle and friendly way.' Teacher commentary and praise as they touch pleases the couples mentioned and helps the less creative with ideas.

4   Partners co-operate, planning their shared play activity, as they now do naturally every week. The profusion of shared activity possibilities, all of which will have been experienced, is a tribute to an excellent programme of physical education.

Friendships Dance

1–2   Partners are challenged to make the final sequences of their Dance programme's final lesson more interesting. Direction changes; being together and apart; some travelling and some dancing on the spot; strong body-shapes contrasts; and, of course, enthusiastic, vigorous and poised participation, are all elements being encouraged by the teacher.

3–6   Pupils now go to their places to dance: (a) the starting stage, dancing and playing alone as a new pupil; (b) the walking, looking at and smiling at others, second stage; (c) responding to a drum beat by making a gentle, friendly contact with someone; and, finally, (d) the partners' planned, shared, repeating pattern of friendly, enjoyable, playful activity.

7–9   Half-watching-half demonstrations with follow-up friendly comments from pupils and the teacher are followed by hands joined to move and sing 'in a big, friendly class circle'.

Games

Introduction to Games for Infant Classes

Individual and team games are part of our national heritage and an essential part of the physical education programme. Skills learned during games lessons lend themselves to being practised away from school, alone or with friends or parents, and are the skills most likely to be used in participating in worthwhile physical and social activities after leaving school – an important, long-term aim in physical education.

Vigorous, whole body activity in the fresh air promotes normal, healthy growth and physical development, stimulating the heart, lungs and big muscle groups, particularly the legs. Games lessons come nearest to demonstrating what we understand by the expression 'children at play' with pupils involved in play-like, exciting, adventurous chasing and dodging as they try to outwit opponents in games and competitive activities. Such close, friendly 'combat' with and against others can help to compensate for the increasingly isolated, over-protected, self-absorbed nature of much of today's childhood.

Games lessons are taught outdoors, in the fresh air, in the playground. For infant classes, the playground 'classroom' can be a netball court, if the school has one, or a painted rectangle, sub-divided into six or eight, 8–10 metre rectangles. A painted rectangle is essential because it:

a contains the whole class in a limited space within which the teacher can see, and be easily seen and heard by, the whole class without straining her or his voice in shouting to be heard over great distances.

b gives the spaces needed for the three activities of the final group practices and games part of the lesson. Each space is normally two adjacent rectangles across the court or one third of the netball court.

c prevents accidents by keeping the class well away from potential hazards such as concrete seats, hutted classrooms, fences or walls, all of which should be several metres outside the games rectangle.

d provides lines which are used in hundreds of ways during the infant years' games programme. Pupils run and jump over; balance on; can be 'safe' on in chasing games; aim at; play new games over; use in limited area 'invent a game or practice' situations; play end to end, two with and two against games; and do side to side relays.

Games will appeal to, and be very popular with the majority of pupils if the pupils are always moving; the games are exciting; nobody is left doing nothing; they are fun to play; there is plenty of action; and if rules prevent quarrels, let the games run smoothly and let everyone have a turn and prevent foul play.

The following monthly lesson plans and accompanying notes aim to provide teachers and schools with a wide variety of material for lesson content, development and progression. Each lesson is repeated three or four times to allow plenty of time for planning, practising, repeating and improving.

The following pages also aim to provide a focus for staffroom togetherness and unity of purpose regarding the programme's aims, content and expectations of standards and levels of achievement.

The Infant School Games Lesson Plan – 30 minutes

Warm-up and Footwork Practices (5 minutes) provide a lively start, put the class in the mood for activity, and aim to improve the quality of the running, jumping, chasing, dodging, marking, and changing speed and direction.

Skills Practices (10 minutes) form the middle part of the lesson, ideally with all using the same implement so that teaching applies to everyone. Infant lessons will include:

- **individual practices** which allow maximum opportunity to improve as pupils practise with ball, bean bag, skipping rope, hoop, quoit, bat or racket and ball.

- **partner practices** to experience the unpredictable behaviour of a ball, for example at different heights, speeds, angles as it does in a game. In co-operative partner practices, partners help each other to master the skills. In competitive partner practices the challenging nature of games, with the testing of skills and wits, and striving to overcome an adversary, are experienced.

Group Practices and Games (15 minutes) are the climax of the lesson, receiving fifteen minutes to allow five minutes for each of the three activities. This important part of the lesson must be given its full time allocation, even if it means cutting other parts short. One of the three activities will always use the implement and the skills practised in the middle of the lesson.

Organisation of the Group Practices and Games Part of the Lesson

At the start of the school year, the class is divided into three mixed groups. They are trained to go and stand in their own starting rectangle within the grids, or thirds of the netball court, when asked 'Please go to your starting places for group activities.' The three sets of implements to be used will have been placed adjacent to, but outside, the enclosed rectangles where they will be used. Balls, bean bags and skipping ropes, for example, are contained within plastic crates to keep them tidy.

The teacher checks that the numbers in each third are correct. If one group has absentees, some pupils are transferred from another group. Then the teacher says, for example, 'Please collect your rope, ball between two, or bean bag between two for your first activity.' When all are standing ready, implement in hand, or beside a partner, the teacher gives a clear explanation of each activity before saying 'Please begin.' The teacher then circulates round the three group practices, giving reminders of the practices and checking that the spacing apart is satisfactory for good practising, and always within the group's own third of the 'playground classroom'.

During the following three lessons of this lesson's development, group activities start with the instruction 'Please go to your starting group places', easily remembered from the previous lesson. They are asked to collect their first activity implement before being told to begin. The teacher circulates round the three different practices or games, reminding them of the practices and main teaching points, progressing the work, giving praise and occasionally presenting a demonstration.

Games equipment. Schools should ensure they have the following:

- sets of 30 of: small balls, medium balls, large balls, beanbags, skipping ropes, playbats, short tennis rackets
- 10 long, 7m skipping ropes for group skipping and for use as 'nets' for tennis and quoits
- 10 rubber quoits
- 6 large 20cm foam balls
- 8 marker cones
- 1 x set Kwik cricket
- playground chalk

A Pattern for Teaching a Games Skill or Practice

Excellent lesson 'pace' is expressed in almost non-stop activity with no bad behaviour stoppages and no 'dead spots' caused by queues, over-long explanations or too many time-consuming demonstrations. The teaching of each of the skills combining to make a games lesson determines the quality of the lesson's pace – a main feature of an excellent physical education lesson.

A typical games lesson with its warm-up and footwork practices, skills practices, and small-sided group practices and games, will have about a dozen skills. Whatever the skill, there is a pattern for teaching it.

1 **Quickly into action**. In a few words, explain the task, and challenge the class to start. 'Can you stand, two big steps apart, and throw and catch the small ball to your partner for a two-handed catch?' If a short demonstration is needed, the teacher can work with a pupil who has been alerted. Class practice should start quickly after the five seconds it took the teacher to make the challenge.

2 **Emphasise the main teaching points, one at a time, while the class is working**. A well-behaved class does not need to be stopped to listen to the next point. 'Hold both hands forward to show your partner where to aim.' 'Watch the ball into your cupped hands.'

3 **Identify and praise good work, while the class is working**. Comments are heard by all; remind the class of key points; and inspire the praised to even greater effort. 'Well done, Sarah and Daniel. You are throwing and catching at the right height and speed, and watching the ball into your hands.'

4 **Teach for individual improvement while class are working**. 'Liam, hold both hands forward to give Charlotte a still target to aim at.' 'Grace and Ali, stand closer. You are too far apart.'

5 **A demonstration can be used**, briefly, to show good quality or an example of what is required. 'Stop everyone, please, and watch how Lucy and Michael let their hands "give" as they receive the ball, to stop it bouncing out again.' Less than twelve seconds later, all resume practising, understanding what 'giving hands' means.

6 **Very occasionally, to avoid taking too much activity time, a short demonstration can be followed by comments**. 'Stop and watch Ahmed and Emily. Tell me what makes their throwing and catching so smooth and accurate.' The class watch about six throws and three or four comments are invited. For example, 'They are nicely balanced with one foot forward.' 'Their hands are well forward, to take the ball early, then give, smoothly and gently.'

7 **Thanks are given to performers and those making helpful comments**. Further practice takes place with reminders of the good things seen and commented on.

Progressing a Games Lesson over 4 or 5 Lessons

Gymnastic activities and dance lessons can begin at a simple level of performing the actions neatly, because they are natural and easy. The challenge for the teacher and class is then to plan and develop movement sequences that link these natural actions together, and refine them by adding 'movement elements' such as changes of speed, direction, shape and tension.

Developing a games lesson is different from the above because the eventual target is the mastery of the specific games skills included in the lesson. Such skills include:

○ good footwork used in stopping, starting, changing direction, chasing after and dodging away from other players

○ sending, receiving and travelling with a ball in invasion, striking/fielding and net games, and controlling other games implements such as skipping ropes, quoits, rackets, hoops and bean bags

○ inventing games with agreed rules in co-operation with a partner or small group. Fairness, safety, lots of action and an understanding of the need for rules are the intended outcomes.

○ playing competitive games as individuals, with partners, and in small-sided games

○ understanding the skills and particular roles of players as they attack and defend in the three types of games.

Often the starting point, practising the new skill, is a problem, because controlling the implement is difficult. Balls, bats, hoops, skipping ropes, rackets, quoits and bean bags behave unpredictably and the teacher has to simplify the planned skills to enable pupils to succeed and progress in subsequent lessons. Reception class pupils, for example, might have to walk beside a partner, handing the bean bag to each other, before progressing to throwing and catching. In a Junior school, 2 versus 1 throwing and catching practice, the teacher can ask the defending pupil in the middle, to be passive, with arms down at sides, not aiming to 'steal' the ball that is being passed, and only keeping between the two passing players to make them move sideways and forwards, into a good space to receive the ball.

The varied skills headings listed, fit neatly into both infant and junior games lessons, with their:

○ footwork practices

○ skills practices, which can include 'invent a game'

○ group practices and small-sided games, which can include 'invent a game' and challenges to suggest ways to improve a game with a new rule, other ways to score, or limits on player movement.

Step by step, revising the previous lesson's work, and introducing only one teaching point at a time, the teacher progresses one of the skills of the lesson, for example:

1　Try the slow overhead pull of the rope as it slides along the ground towards you.

2　Can you travel, running over the sliding rope, one foot after the other? Which is your leading leg?

3　On the spot, try a jump and bounce for each turn of the rope. (Slow '1 and, 2 and' skipping action.)

4　Try slow running over the rope. Use a small, turning wrist action with hands out wide at waist height.

5　Skip from space to space. Then show me skipping in each space.

6　On the spot, try the slow double beat and the quicker single beat. Then show me neat, non-stop skipping.

7　Pretend your group is on a stage, all doing your best skipping.

National Curriculum Requirements for Games –
Key Stage 1: the Main Features

'The Government believes that two hours of physical activity a week, including the National Curriculum for Physical Education and extra-curricular activities, should be an aspiration for all schools. This applies to all key stages.'

Programme of study

Pupils should be taught to:

a travel with, send and receive a ball and other equipment in different ways. Equipment used in the following lessons includes balls of various sizes and textures, bats, rackets, beanbags, quoits, skipping ropes of different lengths, and hoops

b develop these skills for simple net, striking/fielding and invasion-type games. Neat, controlled footwork with changes of speed and direction used to pursue, dodge or simply to give you ample practising room, makes chasing games more exciting and safe

c play simple, competitive net, striking/fielding and invasion-type games that they and others have made, using simple tactics for attacking and defending. From the simplest 'Can you aim at the line between you and your partner and count your good hits to see who is the winner?' to 'Can you invent a simple, 1-against-1 game, using one ball and a part of a line, and using the skills we have just practised?' to 'Can your group of four make up a game, using the large ball and two of the lines around the area?'

At every stage, the pupils will be asked to consider, 'How will you score in your little game? What will be the main rule to make your game fair for everyone? How will your game re-start after a score? Can you think of any extra ways to make the game more exciting?' and, if necessary, 'How can we help to make scoring easier?' (e.g. defending team will be 'passive', not going for the ball).

Attainment target

Pupils should be able to demonstrate that they can:

a select and use skills, actions and ideas appropriately, applying them with co-ordination and control (e.g. throw ball up, jump to catch it, land nicely poised)

b vary, copy, repeat and link skills, actions and ideas in ways that suit the activities (i.e. ample equipment needed to provide an implement each to enable such practising)

c talk about differences between own and others' work and suggest ways to improve their own performance

d recognise and describe the changes that happen to the body during exercise (from increased warmth, perspiration, deep breathing, chest rising and falling, and fatigue, to 'feeling relaxed, calm, happy, good inside, proud, excited').

Main NC headings when considering assessment, progression and expectation

○ **Planning** – in a safe, thoughtful, focused way, thinking ahead to an intended outcome. The set criteria are used and there is evidence of originality and variety

○ **Performing and improving performance** – pupils work hard, concentrating on the main feature of the task, to present a neat, efficient, poised, confident performance, under control

○ **Linking actions** – pupils work harder for longer, smoothly and safely, using space sensibly, and able to remember and repeat the whole sequence successfully from its start right through to its controlled finish

○ **Reflecting and making judgements** to help pupils progress and improve, as they plan again adapting and altering as required, guided by their own and others' comments and judgements.

Year 2 Games Programme

Pupils should be able to:

Autumn	Spring	Summer
1 Respond readily and vigorously to instructions.	**1** Respond immediately and safely, showing a whole-hearted attitude in the pursuit of improved skill.	**1** Show improved ability in running, hurdling, and jumping high and long.
2 Practise, almost non-stop, to improve.	**2** Plan and practise thoughtfully, almost without stopping – repeating, adapting, improving.	**2** Show good control in sending and receiving a ball, alone and with a partner – bat, bowl, throw, roll, serve.
3 Show good space awareness, avoiding others, for continuous, safe, undisturbed practice.	**3** Link movements together with increasing versatility and control, using Games equipment with skill, confidence and enthusiasm.	**3** Continue practising with a wide range of implements – racket and ball, rope, hoop, beanbag, quoit.
4 Run and jump strongly, with good, relaxed arm, leg and upper body carriage, tall and poised.	**4** Demonstrate knowledge and understanding as well as skill in well-planned performances.	**4** Practise hand and racket short tennis over a line or net co-operatively with a partner, and, when ready, competitively, agreeing how to serve, score and keep the game going.
5 Play chasing and dodging games with good footwork, and changes of speed and direction.	**5** Show increasing awareness of ways to receive, send and travel with a ball.	**5** Invent a game in 2s or 4s, in a small area, deciding scoring systems, the main rules, and how to re-start after scoring.
6 Plan to practise a variety of skills with ball, bat, beanbag, hoop, rope, quoit, racket.	**6** Make up and play simple games with little equipment and few, simple rules.	**6** Practise to improve skipping of all kinds, including follow a leader and group skipping with a long rope.
7 Link movements with increasing control, keeping action going to work harder for longer.	**7** Work vigorously to keep warm.	**7** Play 1 v 1, 2 v 2, 3 v 1, 3 v 3, and 4 v 4 competitive games, depending on skill levels, of batting, bowling, fielding; serving, striking, returning.
8 Co-operate with a partner to: send, receive and travel with a ball; rally over net with ball and quoit; lead and follow.	**8** Chase and dodge, changing speed and direction, to avoid being caught.	**8** Link series of simple actions – skip on spot and moving; throw, run, catch; run to field, pick up, throw in; throw to self, bat up, catch, jump high and long.
9 Pass a big ball to partner, then move to a new space for the return pass. Give and go!	**9** Co-operate with a partner to improve skills with ball, beanbag, bat, rope.	**9** Display fair play, honest competition and good sporting behaviour.
10 Play 3 v 1, with the '3' keeping ball from '1' by passing and moving to space for next pass.	**10** Play simple 1 v 1, 2 v 1, 3 v 1 and 2 v 2 games in a limited space, with simple rules and scoring systems.	**10** With partners and in groups, invent and play simple versions of well-known games like tennis and cricket.
11 Make up and play simple games with e.g. one ball, two hoops and a limited area. Decide the main rules, how to score and how to re-start.	**11** Demonstrate skills willingly, and be keen to learn from and use helpful constructive comments made.	**11** Describe what you and others are doing, and make simple judgements on a peformance.
12 Pick out the main features in a demonstration and praise them.		

Year 2

Lesson Plan 1 • 30 minutes
September

Emphasis on: *re-establishing tradition of: (a) immediate responses to instructions; (b) enthusiastic and vigorous participation; (c) safe and sensible sharing of space.*

Warm-up and Footwork Practices
5 minutes

1 Show me that you can run quietly, without following anyone. Lift heels, knees, arms and head, and run straight, not curving. (Unless taught otherwise, children run in an anti-clockwise circle.)

2 Can you use this best, straight running to visit every part of our playground 'classroom' within the four outer lines? Visit the ends, sides, corners and the middle sometimes.

3 When I call 'Stop!' show me how quickly you can respond and stand, balanced on tiptoes, on the nearest line, arms stretched sideways to help your balance.

Skills Practices: with small bats and balls
10 minutes

Individual practices

1 Walk around with ball balanced on bat, near eye level. Now change to gentle batting upwards using wrist action only. What is your best, new year score? Five or more is very good.

2 Throw ball straight up with one hand, let it bounce up, bat it up, catch it with one hand. Repeat.

3 Can you walk around, always looking for good spaces, batting your ball down on to the ground (illustrated)?

Partner practices

1 Can you and your partner keep your ball up in the air between you, using gentle strokes by using your wrists only? (Not elbows or shoulders, which are far too powerful for this neat stroke.)

2 Can you strike the ball up to land between you for a return strike by your partner? Stand only two or three steps apart and keep your best score.

3 One partner bowls underarm with a very slow and low lob for partner to bat back to bowler for catching practice. Have six goes and then change.

Group Practices
15 minutes

Large ball between two

Practise ways to send the ball to your partner, both standing and on the move. How many body parts can send ball quite accurately?

Fours: one bat and ball; half the area

Can you make up a simple batting game, using bat, ball, skittles and lines to 'contain' games? How will you score? How will you be 'out'? How many balls each?

Skipping rope each

Free practice to revise and try out some of the many ways of skipping. On the spot, feet apart or together, or one after the other. Moving in different directions.

Games

Teaching notes and NC guidance
Development over 4 lessons

Warm-up and Footwork Practices

1 Class needs a start-of-year reminder of what 'good running' means or they will return to the noisy, anti-clockwise running in one big circle.

2 Running along straight lines, not curves, enables pupils to visit every part of the teaching space because they are continually coming to an outside line and needing to change direction. Such 'non-following' in physical education gives each child lots of room and time to perform unimpeded.

3 Exercises in listening and responding immediately to the teacher's signals and instructions are important. Poor responders can be made to behave and respond better so that valuable time is not wasted waiting for someone each time.

Skills Practices: with small bats and balls

Individual practices

1 'Performing simple skills safely to join them together with increasing control' satisfies a main requirement within the NC. Balancing, alternate with a little hit upwards, watching the ball closely and using just the right amount of force, is a difficult skill for young pupils.

2 Batting the ball almost straight upwards to let it bounce almost straight upwards for the next hit needs a gentle touch, using a wrist action, not elbow or shoulder.

3 Using the bat like a big hand, pupils now hit the ball down and a little way forwards as they walk forwards, trying to make the bounce up come nicely to where the next step will take them.

Partner practices

1 Standing next to each other, each partner in turn bats the ball straight up between them. The other partner makes the next little hit up. Pupils have to be told to stand 'close enough to touch your partner' so that a vertical (and very gentle) hit is possible.

2 Still close together, they hit the ball gently and straight up, high enough to make it bounce up for the partner to hit up.

3 At 3 metres apart, the bowler aims a 'low and slow' lob to land about 1 metre ahead of the batter to bounce up for a hit at chest height, ideally side-on to the bowler and catcher.

Group practices

Large ball between two

A variety of ways to send (including throwing), receive and travel with a ball is an NC emphasis. The ways pupils receive and control are as important as the sending.

Fours: one bat and ball; half the area

In half of their third of the teaching area, pupils are challenged to 'invent a simple batting game'. They must agree on the style of the game, how to score, how to involve all in the game fairly, and the one main rule that keeps the game going and fair.

Skipping rope each

Free practice will be as varied and challenging as teacher commentary and praise can make it. Quiet, neat footwork; good rope control; and varied directions and speeds are encouraged.

Year 2

Lesson Plan 2 • 30 minutes
October

Emphasis on: *(a) practising, almost non-stop, to improve; (b) practising good footwork, including dodging and chasing; (c) practising varied ball skills.*

Warm-up and Footwork Practices
5 minutes

1   Run, practising little side steps to avoid others coming towards you. In a side step, one foot goes out to the side instead of forwards, to put you on to a new line, still facing the same way.

2   Five points tag. All have five points to start with. When touched you lose one of your points. (N.B. No dangerous pushing. Touch gently.)

Skills Practices: with a large or medium ball
10 minutes

Individual practices

1   Walk, throwing the ball just above your head and then catching it. Keep your fingers spread, thumbs back, fingers around the sides of the ball.

2   Bounce the ball using your finger-tips, left and right hands, on the spot, and weaving in and out of the others.

3   Dribble the ball like a footballer, keeping it close. When I call 'Stop!' see how quickly you can control the ball by placing a foot on top of the ball, to make it still.

Partner practices

1   About 3 metres apart only, throw a two-handed pass to your partner and move sideways into a space for the return pass, still only 3 metres apart. Pass; move; receive.

2   Shadow dribbling, one ball. Leader shows partner favourite ways to dribble, using feet or hands. After six touches, change over and see if the follower can copy the routine exactly.

Group Practices
15 minutes

Quoits: with a partner; 1 v 1

Long rope 'net' tied between chairs. Play quoits and try to score by landing quoit on a partner's side for a point. Decide how to start, how many points to a game, and any other rules to help the game.

Large ball among four: 3 v 1

'Wandering ball' with three of group on outside of big chalk circle passing the ball across the circle, bypassing and outwitting the one in the circle (illustrated). Keep changing one in centre who works hard to intercept the ball.

Partners: with a hoop each

Stand at opposite side of court from partner. Bowl hoop to pass each other and go to partner's line. Keep close to and in control of your hoop. Now can you show me another good partner practice you like?

Games

Teaching notes and NC guidance
Development over 4 lessons

Warm-up and Footwork Practices

1   To give continuous practice of meeting others, the side step is done in one third of the teaching space, to bring everyone close together. The running is at half speed to let pupils focus on and do the side steps in safety.

2   In five points tag, the class is asked to dodge away from chasers, not race away at high speed. 'Dodging' means changing direction; side stepping; and making sudden changes of speed, including stopping suddenly. The game is stopped every 15 seconds to let the teacher check on 'Who were the best dodgers with 5 points still? Who were the best chasers, catching 3 or more?'

Skills Practices: with a large or medium ball

Individual practices

1   The throw to above the head is performed from a high position at head height with the ball in both hands, arms slightly bent, and fingers pointing upwards. Hands receive with a little 'give' each time, and eyes watch the ball closely.

2   In bouncing, basketball fashion, we use the fingertips and a wrist action, up and down where you stand, and forwards and down when travelling. Use left and right hands to avoid others coming towards you.

Partner practices

1   The two-handed chest pass starts in front of the passer's chest with hands higher than elbows. Ball is pushed to partner's chest height for a catch where the arms 'give' to stop ball rebounding away. The move sideways to a new space to receive the next pass is one of the most important moves in invasion games. 'Pass, then move!' will continually be said during games lessons from now on. This movement is needed by a team to advance itself and the ball towards the opponents' goal line.

2   Shadow dribbling trains the leader to think about and plan a short sequence, and trains the follower to observe and be able to repeat the sequence.

Group Practices

Quoits: with a partner; 1 v 1

In competitive, 1-against-1 quoits, the 'net' is a long rope tied between chairs or higher objects, ideally at chest height so that the throw has to be high enough to 'let the quoit see over the net'. A point is scored if the quoit lands on the ground. Pairs have to agree how to start or serve; ways to score; and one main rule designed to keep the game going and fair.

Large ball among four: 3 v 1

In 'wandering ball' or piggy in the middle around a chalk circle of 2 metres diameter, the 3 must stay outside the circle, and the 1 must stay inside it. If the game keeps breaking down with few passes being made, the 1 can be asked to be passive, keeping arms by the sides, to make passing easier.

Partners: with a hoop each

Bowling the hoops to change places, line to line, is done at a walking pace, keeping beside your hoop, not pushing it far ahead.

Lesson Plan 3 • 30 minutes
November

Emphasis on: *(a) linking movements with increasing control to keep the action going longer; (b) making up and playing simple games.*

Warm-up and Footwork Practices
5 minutes

1 Change between easy jogging and bursts of sprinting. Jog when you are near others. Sprint when you see a good space. Arms and heels are low in jogging, lifted up when sprinting.

2 Chain tag with four couples starting off as chasers. When someone is caught, he or she joins the pair that caught them. When the chain grows to four, it separates into two chains of one couple each who then continue to chase. Winner is last one caught.

Skills Practices: with a skipping rope
10 minutes

Individual practices

1 Practise the slow overhead pull and the easy step over as the rope slides along the ground towards you. Hand action is very small.

2 Now skip on the move with a sort of running action. Which is your leading leg?

Partner practices

Stand where you can see each other easily. A will skip for about six travelling counts and stop. B will skip for about six counts and stop. Can you include a variety of directions and try to have one of the pair on the move at all times? Your working–resting partner skipping will be interesting if you can do some opposites (e.g. forwards, backwards; feet apart, together).

Group Practices
15 minutes

Large ball among four: 2 v 2

Play 2 against 2 in half of your area, and score by bouncing ball in one of the choice of hoops. Can you agree one main rule to help keep the game fair? What other way to score can you think of to give more goals?

Long skipping rope among four

Two swing rope low, for others to jump (illustrated). While learning, do not swing the long rope over-head. Come in to the rope when it is swinging away from you. Leave the rope left when it is swinging to the right.

Beanbag among three: 2 v 1

Piggy in the middle with the two with the beanbag moving to a space to receive from partner. Middle person tries to intercept by spreading arms and legs wide. Use two-handed pass, then move to a new space, ready.

Games

Teaching notes and NC guidance
Development over 4 lessons

Warm-up and Footwork Practices

1 The teacher can demonstrate easy jogging with arms and heels lower than normal, lively running, an upright body, and with a nice, steady rhythm. Short bursts of sprinting for 4 to 6 metres through a space has rapid short strides, a high lift of heels and knees, and a body inclined forwards.

2 In the chasing and dodging chain tag, chasers must touch gently and safely, and not push the dodgers to catch them. Encourage the dodgers to try side steps, direction changes and sudden changes of speed to evade chasers, never high speed running away.

Skills Practices: with a skipping rope

Individual practices

1 All practise the slow, overhead pull to remind themselves of the easy, wide hand action and the physically easy step over the rope.

2 The slow step over the rope becomes a quicker run over it as the class try to skip 'on the move', noting which leg is leading. This one foot after the other is easier, physically, than skipping on the spot with feet together. 'Easier' means you can keep going and keep warm as we move into colder weather.

Partner practices

Resting and working; watching and doing; alternate skipping gives pupils a rest and challenges them to plan a sequence that has variety (and quality, we hope) of actions, leg shapes, directions and speeds. 'Someone working at all times' means a smooth transition from one performer to the partner, with excellent timing.

Group Practices

Large ball among 4: 2 v 2

The competitive, 2 versus 2, with one ball in half of their third, requires the passing pair to 'Pass, then move to a new space to receive the next pass' or they will never advance themselves or the ball, because you may not run carrying the ball. To make this feature succeed, it might be necessary to ask the two defenders to be passive, never going for the ball when it is being passed, but able to intercept shots.

Long skipping rope among four

A 4-metres long rope is swung low, from side to side, vigorously. (Not overhead to start with.) Group has turns at swinging the rope, then trying to come in to skip. They should aim to come in to skip along the line on the ground where the rope touches each time. Beginners usually jump too early at a point where the rope is well off the ground.

Beanbag among three: 2 v 1

The pair with the beanbag are asked to wait until the receiving partner has moved sideways into a space before throwing to that partner. They must not throw it over the head of the one in the middle. If this game is being badly done with few successful passes and catches, ask the one in the middle to be passive and not challenge for the beanbag.

Year 2

Lesson Plan 4 • 30 minutes
December

Emphasis on: *(a) near-continuous, lively action to become and to stay warm; (b) strong leg activity, which increases winter warmth.*

Warm-up and Footwork Practices
5 minutes

1 Follow the leader, where the leader uses a simple repeating pattern, e.g. walk 6, jog 6, jump with feet together for 6. Change over and see if follower can remember and repeat it all.

2 'Line safe tag', where the six chasers can catch you if you are not on a line, i.e. on a line is safe, untouchable. Those caught take a coloured band and become chasers. If dodgers are staying too long on their lines, teacher calls 'All move!'

Skills Practices: with a beanbag
10 minutes

Individual practices

1 Jog forwards, throwing up and forwards a little way with one hand, and catching with two hands.

2 Throw low (chest height), throw medium (head height), throw high (as high as can be caught reliably), and try to do this on the move to keep warm.

3 Stand. Throw beanbag to one side or the other; in front of you; or behind you. Can you move quickly to catch it with two hands? Throw it high enough to give you time to get there.

Partner practices

1 Jog around, side by side, passing the bag like a rugby ball with long straight arms swinging across from side to side. Throw and catch with two hands. Aim just in front of your partner.

2 Stand 3 metres apart. Throw with one hand, move to a new space and catch with two hands. Hold your hands forwards to show your partner a target to aim at. Pass; move; receive, moving sideways and forwards to maintain the 2–3-metre distance.

3 Stand very close. Throw above partner's head for a high jump up to catch at full stretch with one or both hands (illustrated).

Group Practices
15 minutes

Free practice: with choice of ropes, hoops, balls, quoits, bats and balls
Choose something you can use in a lively, vigorous way, using large body actions, as you share the space sensibly.

Beanbag among four: team passing; 2 against 2, or 3 against 1
Play 2 v 2, if good skill level; 3 v 1 if not so good. Keep close enough to give partner an easy 2–3-metre pass. Three good passes can equal a goal.

Partners with a large ball
Keep on the move to show me how you can carry, send and receive your ball with lots of success, keeping going, almost non-stop, to keep warm.

Games

Teaching notes and NC guidance
Development over 4 lessons

Warm-up and Footwork Practices

1 To inspire an instant response, the class can be asked to follow the leader performing the teacher's suggested, simple, short sequence with its walk, jog and jump, always looking for good spaces to lead your partner through. When 'pattern' is understood the class can be invited to keep the same simple sequence or adapt it to one of their own planning. Each part must be kept short.

2 Because December can be very cold we do not want too many instances of inactive loitering on the 'safe' lines. After 20 seconds, the teacher checks on who were the best dodgers, still not caught, and changes the chasers over.

Skills Practices: with a beanbag

Individual practices

1 Because it is easy to catch and hold, a beanbag is a good implement for cold weather throwing and catching, as it does not roll or bounce away from you. The little throw forwards is to about head height and just ahead of you.

2 Still jogging while practising to keep warm, still throwing with one hand and catching with two, pupils feel the different amounts of force needed to make it go 'Low; medium; higher'.

3 A standing throw up and to one side or to the front is followed by a quick move to a position where you can catch the beanbag while standing still with hands forwards and cupped – another example of 'simple skills joined together'.

Partner Practices

1 In jogging side by side, emphasise that your body is facing forwards normally with long, low arms swinging from side to side, with the hands around the sides of the ball. (Children often run with their whole body moving sideways, not facing to the front.)

2 This 'Pass, then move!' practice is one of the most important in Games. The move, usually to one side and forwards, into a space, means that you are available to receive the next pass in a space, and the ball is advancing towards the opponents' line.

3 Jumping partner must wait until ball starts to come down before he or she jumps up to meet it at full stretch, then land, nicely balanced, with feet astride.

Group Practices

Free practice: with a choice of ropes, hoops, balls, quoits, bats and balls

In free practice in December, the main feature must be the vigorous action asked for, to keep warm. Ideally, whole-body actions, able to be repeated, non-stop, are being planned and practised, e.g. running style skipping with high knee raising.

Beanbag among four: team passing; 2 against 2, or 3 against 1

Competitive 2 v 2, or 3 v 1, team passing with a beanbag, gives excellent practice in the important 'Pass, then move for the next pass – in a space you have made by moving.'

Partners with a large ball

The three-part sequence asks for a controlled carry, a sending that is accurate and neat, and a receiving that looks easy because the receiver is in the right place and ready.

Lesson Plan 5 • 30 minutes
January

Emphasis on: *(a) engaging vigorously in activities to keep warm; (b) co-operating with a partner to improve and extend skills.*

Warm-up and Footwork Practices
5 minutes

1 Follow your leader, who will show you two or three lively actions to warm up the big muscles, particularly the legs. Can you copy these actions precisely? (Look out for, comment on and encourage jogging, sprinting, jumping, bouncing, hopping, skipping, leaping.)

2 Couples tag. Four couples start off as chasers. When one of the pair touches a dodger, the caught boy or girl changes place with the one who caught them to form a new chasing couple.

Skills Practices: with a large ball – 10 minutes

Individual practices

1 Carry ball in both hands like a rugby player. Run around and when I call 'Change!' place your ball down like a rugby player scoring a try, and pick up a different ball. Continue running and listening for my signal to 'Change!'

2 Throw ball up and forwards a short distance ahead of you. Run to catch with two hands near eye level.

Partner practices

1 Jog, side by side, passing the ball, rugby fashion, a short distance in front of your partner to let him or her run and meet it each time. Use two hands and a lot of care.

2 Make two-handed chest and bounce passes to each other at about 3 metres apart. After every pass, move sideways and forwards to a new space to receive the return pass. Pass; move; receive.

Group Practices
15 minutes

Skipping rope each

On the spot, practise the slow double beat of feet for every turn of the rope, and the quicker single beat. Skip on the move and show me your best style of non-stop skipping. Direction changes are interesting.

Five large balls among group of ten

Five with balls are dodging away from the others, who are trying to touch a ball to gain it. Rugby style game with ball carriers allowed to run, carrying in both hands. Touch ball gently, not the person.

Large ball among four: 2 v 2; half pitch

Invent a 'three lives' game with one pair having three attacks to score. After defence steal ball three times, teams change duties. Decide how to score; one main rule to keep game going; and how to re-start after a goal.

Games

Teaching notes and NC guidance
Development over 4 lessons

Warm-up and Footwork Practices

1 In mid-winter the class can be told about this first energetic activity while still in the classroom. Partners can be arranged and the action can start immediately they reach the play area. Stoppages for explanations or demonstrations will be kept to a minimum, and most of the teaching and praising takes place while the class is moving.

2 Couples tag keeps pupils moving vigorously in pursuit or dodging. It also keeps them thinking as the catcher breaks away from the pair and the newly caught pupil joins on. The game is stopped every 30 seconds or so to check on 'Who are the good dodgers, not caught at all?' and to introduce new chasers.

Skills Practices: with a large ball

Individual practices

1 Ball is carried in both hands with straight arms hanging low in front of you. With the rhythm of the running, the ball is gently swung from side to side. On 'Change!' ensure that the ball is placed, not dropped, with downward hands pressure, on to ground.

2 Throw up and forwards a short distance. Make throw high enough to allow a catch near eye level with two hands. Be sensible about the space you throw in to. Avoid others.

Partner practices

1 Emphasise low carry of ball in front of you. Arms swing from side to side naturally. Keep body facing forwards while running, but twist upper body to face partner as you pass ball just ahead of him or her, high enough for a good mid-chest catch.

2 Chest pass is aimed at partner's chest. Bounce pass is aimed at ground about 1 metre in front of partner. After every pass, move to a new space, but still only about 3 metres apart. If 'Pass, then move! Give, then go! Pass, run to a space!' is emphasised at this age, the quality of team play, now and in the junior school, will be greatly improved.

Group Practices

Skipping rope each

Give them something to think about and plan while skipping on the spot or moving. Single- and double-beat foot action on the spot for slower or quicker skipping, with one or two bounces for each rope turn. On the move can be with feet together, or like running with one foot after the other.

Five large balls among group of ten

Rugby ball touch is helped by pupils being allowed to run, holding the ball in a rugby style. Teacher can add interest by calling 'Change!' when all the carriers must put the ball on the ground and let the other half of the group become the dodgers.

Large ball among four: 2 v 2; half pitch

Three lives' games played in one direction only have the same attackers and defenders until the defenders steal possession thrice. This allows two little games to be played in the one third. Teams need to decide the one main rule, the scoring method, and how to re-start after a score.

Lesson Plan 6 • 30 minutes
February

Emphasis on: *(a) showing increasing control over own movement; (b) linking movements to demonstrate increasing versatility.*

Warm-up and Footwork Practices
5 minutes

1 Can you run and jump high, run and jump long over the lines and show me the difference? (High: at medium speed, rocking up on take-off foot, with leading bent knee reaching up. Long: at speed, with long, straight, leading leg well forwards.)

2 Teacher's space tag. Teacher and four helpers 'guard' the middle third of the playground, touching the remainder to prevent them scoring a point for a clear run to opposite side of third. Four helpers are changed over often.

Skills Practices: with a skipping rope
10 minutes

Individual practices

1 Choose one way to skip that you find easy. Can you all keep going for a whole minute, starting from... now!

2 Can you link together a way of skipping on the spot with one on the move, and keep alternating them?

Partner practices

1 Place ropes on ground, side by side, about 1 metre apart. Can you make up a little balancing sequence along the ropes as a pair? (For example, one or both hands joined, balancing sideways, forwards or backwards; or facing in different directions.)

2 Watch your partner doing a favourite piece of skipping. Tell your partner what you liked about it. Change.

Group Practices
15 minutes

Large ball between two

Can you invent a 1 against 1, simple game, using one ball and part of a line? How will you score? What is main rule to keep game going? How will you re-start after a score? (For example, 1 v 1, to hand or foot dribble to cross line.)

Partners with rope each

Play follow the leader, where the leader, 3 metres ahead, demonstrates at least two actions for a partner to copy (illustrated). Watch your leader's feet, together or apart; and actions, walking, running, bouncing; and the directions.

Hoop 'safe' tag with eight hoops

Three chasers wearing bands chase to touch the remainder, when they are not 'safe' in a hoop. Those who are caught take a band and become extra chasers. If dodgers 'hide' too long in hoops, teacher calls 'All move!' Gentle touches by chasers. No hard, dangerous pushing.

Games

Teaching notes and NC guidance
Development over 4 lessons

Warm-up and Footwork Practices

1   For unimpeded, safe, continuous practice, pupils should be reminded to 'visit every part of the playground space, never following anyone' and not run in an anti-clockwise circle.

2   Because dodgers are running towards one another across the middle third, they must do so with great care to avoid head-on bumps. Dodgers should be using clever footwork such as direction changes and side steps, and not racing flat out.

Skills Practices: with a skipping rope

Individual practices

1   Easy skipping includes the slow overhead pull and the step over the rope sliding along the ground towards you; running action skipping with one foot leading over the rope; skipping on the spot, slowly, with a double beat of the feet for every swing over of the rope. (Jump and bounce.)

2   Progression in Physical Education includes moving on from simple and isolated movements to making short sequences of linked movements. Here we want skipping on the spot linked to skipping on the move.

Partner practices

1   The words 'balancing sequence', which is the challenge here, mean that more than one way to balance must be planned and practised. One could be with hands joined, one without a join; facing same way could alternate with facing opposite ways.

2   Watching and commenting on a partner demonstration trains pupils in observing the elements of movement. What actions? What use of body parts? What directions? What speed? Saying something about it trains them in reflecting and evaluating, which are important requirements within the NC.

Group Practices

Large ball between two

In a specified, limited area, pupils are challenged to 'invent a competitive, 1 against 1 game'. They have to plan, decide and agree on the nature of the game; how to score within it; what is the one main rule; and how to restart after a goal or point has been scored.

Partners with rope each

The follow-the-leader skipping sequence must have at least two parts to be a sequence, featuring linked actions. Apart from quality, of course, a good sequence includes variety and contrast, e.g. feet together, going sideways quickly, then running feet going forwards slowly.

Hoop 'safe' tag with eight hoops

In hoop 'safe' tag, coloured bands are placed on the ground for the newly caught to pick up and wear as they join the other chasers. Particularly if the weather is cold, the dodgers should be told to 'Linger seldom. Move often' to keep warm and give chasers some activity in pursuing.

Year 2

Lesson Plan 7 • 30 minutes
March

Emphasis on: *(a) varied activities possible with a hoop; (b) demonstrating enthusiastically when asked and watching others' demonstrations with interest and helpful comments.*

Warm-up and Footwork Practices
5 minutes

1 Run quietly, following no-one. When I call 'Change!' change direction by pushing hard with one foot to stop your forwards movement and to make you go another way. Right foot firmly pressed on to ground pushes you off to the left, to run facing a new direction.

2 All-against-all tag, trying not to be caught by others. No hard, dangerous pushing. Touch gently. (Teacher checks best number caught by chasers, and fewest times caught by dodgers.) A sudden direction change is a good dodge.

Skills Practices: with hoops
10 minutes

Individual practices

1 Place all hoops on ground, well spaced out. Run and jump over some hoops and quickly step in and out of some hoops. Pretend some are obstacles and some are stepping stones. When I call 'Stop!' show me how quickly you can find a hoop to stand in. (Repeat.)

2 Can you walk forwards, either bowling your hoop, or doing low, two-handed little throws and catches? Share the space sensibly and don't bump or throw towards others.

3 There are many ways to skip using a hoop, including skipping around it, while on the ground; using one or two hands, forwards and back, side to side, or diagonally; swinging low; or overhead like a skipping rope. Show me what you can do.

Group Practices
15 minutes

Partners, with a quoit: 1 against 1

Make the quoit go over a long rope 'net' tied between chairs or netball posts (illustrated). Decide how to start and score; one main rule to keep game going; and how many points in a game.

Hoop each

Try spinning the hoop on the ground, ankle, wrist or waist. Jog beside your hoop, bowling gently with one hand across top of hoop. Can you spin the hoop to make it come back to you?

Large ball among four: 2 v 2; end line touch

Play in half of your area with several ways agreed to score, e.g. touch end line; bounce in one of hoops in the corners; pass to partner on end line. Decide a main rule to keep game going, and how to re-start.

Games

Teaching notes and NC guidance
Development over 4 lessons

Warm-up and Footwork Practices

1   Pupils have been changing direction in every Games lesson, but probably without thinking about the technique involved. Here we are consciously stopping the forward movement by pressing down hard on one foot which also then sends us off with a strong push into the new direction. A lean of the upper body into the new line is helpful.

2   In all-against-all tag, encourage practice of sudden direction changes to evade a chaser following or coming towards you. For safety's sake, insist on 'Gentle touching only so that no-one is knocked down and hurt.'

Skills Practices: with hoops

Individual practices

1   All 30 hoops being used in the lesson are well spaced out, with ten in each third. Some are placed just close enough to act as 'stepping stones'. A rhythmic pattern is possible. 'Jump over; jump over; step and step and step.'

2   In bowling, walk beside your hoop with your fingers across it, pointing away from you, just below the top. Pull with your hand to try to roll it forwards. In throwing and catching, with both hands wrapped around the hoop, close together, the hands open and close, keeping some contact throughout.

3   Skipping with a slow, short, one-handed swing from side to side is like skipping over a low rope swinging from side to side, and is the easiest to start with, before progressing on to two-handed swing overhead. Two bounces of the feet to each rope swing are recommended.

Group Practices

Partners, with a quoit: 1 against 1

In competitive, 1-against-1 quoits, you score if the quoit lands on the ground on your opponent's side of the rope 'net', which is at head height. One hand is used for throwing and two are used for catching. Some chalk marks for the side of each little 'court' are recommended, to contain the game.

Hoop each

Free practice with a hoop allows more time to practise the skills performed or seen earlier in the lesson and to try out some of the teacher's challenges. 'Can you...?'

Large ball among four

Played in half of a third of the teaching space, 2 v 2 with a large ball aims to encourage each pair to keep possession and to try to advance themselves and the ball to score in ways that they agree. More ways to score make the defending pair space apart more to cover, for example, the end line and the two hoops. Spreading the defenders gives the attackers more room and more chances to score. In this game we hope that the players will decide: how to score, often using more than one way; how to re-start after a score; the one main rule that helps to keep the game going.

Lesson Plan 8 • 30 minutes
April

Emphasis on: *(a) showing good planning in safe, appropriate solutions to tasks; (b) demonstrating good control over body, good sharing of space, and good footwork to be in the right place at the right time.*

Warm-up and Footwork Practices
5 minutes

1   Can you mix quick walking, easy jogging and short bursts of sprinting as you use the whole playground carefully and safely? In jogging, heels and arms are carried low. In your sprints, lift heels and knees strongly.

2   Count how many two-footed jumps you need to cross from one side line to the opposite side line. Use your arms strongly to pull you far forwards. Swing them forwards, then back with a bend of the knees, then swing them forwards and spring from both feet.

Skills Practices: with short-tennis rackets and ball
10 minutes

Individual practices

1   Can you bounce the ball continuously up from your racket? Use a gentle wrist action with racket held near eye level.

2   Can you bounce your ball continuously down on to the ground? Try this standing, then slowly moving forwards, still using the wrist action only. No hard hitting with elbow or shoulder.

3   Throw ball up straight to let it bounce up. Hit it up, let it bounce, catch it with non-hitting hand and start again. What is your best score of controlled hitting and catching?

Partner practices

1   Throw ball to partner who strikes it back for an easy catch. Hit it gently and change over after five catches.

2   Both with a racket now, can you very gently keep the ball bouncing once only, between hits, as you hit low and slow to each other? Start by dropping the ball, letting it bounce up, then sending it. Stand about 4–5 metres apart only, and be gentle.

Group Practices
15 minutes

Ten hoops on ground

Invent a chasing and dodging game, using the hoops and keeping inside your own area. Chasers wear bands. Decide the main rule, how players are caught, what to do when caught.

Short-tennis racket each

Practise by yourself to improve your ball and racket control. You can practise on the spot, hitting up, down or a mixture. Moving, you can hit up, down and from side to side.

Large ball among four

Team passing with 3 against 1. The 3 try to keep the ball and make passes. 1 tries to 'steal' the ball by vigorous chasing after the ball. 1 can be passive if passing is not good and needs help.

Games

Teaching notes and NC guidance
Development over 4 lessons

Warm-up and Footwork Practices

1   'Easy' jogging is done with an upright body, small steps, arms and heels carried low, and is easier than quick walking. The sprinting strides are rapid, with hands and heels carried higher, and are tiring and space consuming, so should be done in short bursts through spaces where others are not impeded.

2   A series of standing, two-footed jumps is performed with each jump starting at the place where the previous one landed. Feet apart with toes turned in slightly; a long arm swing forwards, then back with a knee bend, and forwards strongly with the dynamic stretch of the legs; and a low layout in flight, all help the jump to be as long as possible.

Skills Practices: with short-tennis rackets and ball

Individual practices

1   Racket is held near its face, not near the end of its handle, to give better control, and it is held near the chest so that the ball can be watched closely.

2   Because the racket is springy, pupils do not need to apply much force when batting the ball down to bounce up to waist height for the next hit down. We want them to 'feel' how much or how little force is needed. Beginners usually hit too hard.

3   Throwing up; letting bounce; hitting straight up; and catching are another example of 'performing simple skills and joining them together with increasing control', as required within the NC.

Partner practices

1   If ball is bounced about 1 metre in front of batter and comes up to just above waist height, the batter has an easy return to the bowler, whose hands should be cupped and forwards, ready.

2   In hitting very gently to each other, pupils should again aim to bounce the ball 1 metre in front of partner to give him or her the best possible chance to return it. 'Low and slow' to land for an easy return, ideally from partner's forehand, is the aim.

Group Practices

Ten hoops on ground

With ten inventing and playing a chasing and dodging game, the teacher might initially suggest three chasers wearing bands who can catch you if you are not in a hoop, 'safe' and untouchable. This will give the game a start from which other suggestions will follow from the pupils, e.g. when caught, take a band and become a chaser; 'hiding' in the hoop to be no more than 5 seconds long.

Short-tennis racket each

Racket skills are the most difficult and seldom practised away from school. Personal practice aims to reinforce the work done earlier in the lesson with individual coaching by the teacher.

Large ball among four

Team passing, 3 against 1, is a most important practice for our traditional invasion/running games, such as netball, football, hockey and basketball, to encourage running to a space to be available for a return pass, well away from opponents.

Lesson Plan 9 • 30 minutes
May

Emphasis on: *(a) running, jumping, throwing and skipping; (b) practising to improve performance; (c) dependence on a partner to provide the unpredictable situations so often found in Games*

Warm-up and Footwork Practices
5 minutes

1 Follow your leader who will show you some actions as you run and jump. For example, hurdling, scissors jumping, long and high jumps, and two-footed take-off long jumps.

2 Side-line sprints. Couples stand side by side down the centre of the area. On the signal 'Go!' each sprints to the nearer side line, touches it with a foot and races back to touch partner's hand. A signal 'Four!' or 'Six!', for example, will start a race where pupils sprint to the line and touch it four or six times.

Skills Practices — with a small ball

Individual practices

1 Throw up and catch with two hands at eye level. Now do the same thing, walking and keeping an eye on the ball.

2 Walk forwards, throwing ball up to bounce in front of you. Catch it after the bounce.

3 Can you walk, batting the ball down on to the ground with left and right hands?

Partner practices

1 One partner throws straight for other to catch. Second partner bounces it back. Change over after six.

2 Roll ball for partner to ground, field, pick up and roll back.

3 Stand on opposite sides of a line, about 3 metres from the line. Throw, aiming to hit the line and give partner a catch.

Group Practices
15 minutes

Partners: skittle and a small ball

Bowl to bounce up to hit skittle (illustrated). Partner is wicket keeper who throws or rolls ball back. Have six goes each and change over, keeping your own best score. Can you work out where a 'good length bounce' would land?

Partners: skipping rope each

Can you show me some examples of what we might call 'partner skipping'? You can use own rope and follow the leader, or watch each other's favourite practice. You can try to skip together, using one rope only.

Hand tennis over line or rope 'net'

Serve by dropping ball, letting it bounce up, and then striking it to land on partner's side of net. Decide the one main rule to keep the game fair and going. How many points in a game before changing ends?

Teaching notes and NC guidance
Development over 4 lessons

Warm-up and Footwork Practices

1   May is an appropriate month for using athletics terminology and explaining and showing, for example, hurdling, scissors jumping, and long and high jumping. In hurdling over lines approached from the front, we swing up and down with a straight leading leg and a trailing leg that lifts out and to the side, then forwards. A scissors jump from an angle swings the nearer leg up and over the line.

2   In side-line sprints, everyone starts on the signal. They must touch their own side line and their own partner. Cheating must be looked out for and strongly objected to, so that the winners are the true winners.

Skills Practices: with a small ball

Individual practices

1   Class can all stand, throwing and catching with two hands at eye level, so that teacher can check hand positions and height thrown. If this is satisfactory, they practise on the move, with well-cupped hands and eyes looking closely at the ball.

2   A throw up and forwards, with a swing back and forwards with a long arm, aims to go just high enough and far enough forwards for the next bounce to come up nicely ahead of you for a catch.

3   Continuous batting downwards, 'as in basket-ball', is usually done well by this age group, and is easier with a hand than with a bat or racket. A gentle wrist action is all that is needed.

Partner practices

1   At a distance apart of 3 metres, one throws straight to the partner's outstretched hands in front of chest with a long underarm aiming action. The other partner throws a bounce return with ball starting high above the shoulder, and aiming to land it 1 metre in front of partner, for a chest-height catch.

2   Still 3 metres apart, they roll ball for partner to crouch to field with both hands behind the ball, with fingers facing down.

3   Aiming to hit a line between you and your partner is done with a high starting position with ball above shoulder.

Group Practices

Partners: skittle and a small ball

Bowler aims underarm to land in front of wicket skittle to bounce up to hit it. The many which miss this difficult target will be fielded by the wicket keeper who rolls ball back to the bowler.

Partners: skipping rope each

Year 2 partner skipping produces a most interesting variety of work, as the pupils approach the end of their year. The work deserves to be demonstrated as a way of expanding the class repertoire, and the teacher's repertoire. Skipping together, using one rope only, is now achievable by some.

Hand tennis over line or rope 'net'

For this competitive 1-against-1 hand tennis game over a long rope 'net', they need to agree on: how to serve; how to score; and any allowances to make to keep the game going and fair.

Year 2

Lesson Plan 10 • 30 minutes
June

Emphasis on: *(a) variety from individual, partner and group activities; (b) variety from running, skipping, throwing and striking a ball; (c) variety from planning, doing, reflecting and commenting.*

Warm-up and Footwork Practices
5 minutes

1 With a partner, run side by side at the same speed. Each has a turn at setting the rhythm of the running. Run in good style, with good lifting of heels and knees, and with whole body 'straight ahead'.

2 Jumping alternately, see how few standing long jumps your partner and you need to take you from side line to opposite side line. One jumps and stands still in landing place. Two starts behind toe line of one and does his or her standing, two-footed long jump. Count how many (or few) jumps you needed. Try to improve on the way back by really driving hard and long into your strong leap.

Skills Practices: with a skipping rope
10 minutes

Individual practices

1 Can you link together two or three ways of skipping, including one on the spot and one on the move?

2 Choose one way you enjoy skipping and find easy to keep going. Let me see if the whole class can be brilliant and keep going for a minute. Ready?... Begin!

Partner practices

1 With ropes placed parallel on the ground, can you make up a little balancing sequence along the ropes, as a pair (e.g. side by side or facing each other; one or both hands joined; balance walk forwards, sideways or backwards)?

2 Can you remind each other of some examples of the 'partner skipping' you tried last month? Practise again and try to do something using one rope only.

Group Practices
15 minutes

Groups of four: short-tennis racket or small bat and ball

Two with two tennis over a long rope 'net' tied between chairs. Co-operate to keep a long rally going and keep your best score without a stoppage.

Skipping rope each

Can your whole group practise to show the class a group demonstration of varied skipping – ones, pairs, on the spot and moving, fast and slow, feet together and apart?

Large ball among four in half of area

Can you invent a game for four players, using one ball and the lines around your area? How will you score? What will be your main rule to keep the game fair and going?

Games

Teaching notes and NC guidance
Development over 4 lessons

Warm-up and Footwork Practices

1 Partners running at the same 'cruising' speed should 'feel' the repeating rhythm that is being quietly sounded out by their feet. It should be slow enough to allow a good lifting of knees, heels, arms and head. Keep together, one, two, three, four!

2 In a standing-start broad jump, start with feet slightly apart with toes turned in a little way. Swing both arms forwards high, back with a good knees bend, and forwards hard as you do your reach into your long jump. Pull both feet forwards to land.

Skills Practices: with a skipping rope

Individual practices

1 Skipping on the spot and on the move mixes the more demanding actions on the spot with the physically easier ones while on the move. We can challenge pupils, 'Can you skip with feet together then moving one after the other?' or 'Can you turn the rope to the front while you travel backwards?' or 'Can you include one quick jump for each turn, then the slower two jumps for each turn?'

2 Skipping inspires leg-muscle action, which inspires heart and lungs action, leading to improved fitness. Many primary-school children express an interest in becoming fitter and they can test themselves by trying to keep going for a minute's skipping, which is something they can then practise at home.

Partner practices

1 Ask pupils to try some of the many ways that a pair can join for balancing with a support. As well as both facing the same way, they can have one going forwards, one going backwards. Tell them to 'Feel for the rope with each foot before putting your weight down. Feel for it. Do not look down for it.'

2 Partner skipping can include: following the leader; one watching, the other copying; a mirroring sequence that changes after an agreed number of repetitions; or the difficult pair skipping with only one rope, held by one or both.

Group Practices

Groups of four: short-tennis racket or small bat and ball

Co-operative tennis over a low rope 'net' to 'Find your best score as a group. Can you keep going for six good hits?' Ask them to move early to be in position for the return hit, ideally in a 'side-on' position. Start by dropping the ball for a good bounce up to hit.

Skipping rope each

Emphasise that each rope group will give a demonstration to show variety, quality, and excellent shared use of space, and to increase the class skipping repertoire. Look out for and comment on: on the spot and moving; different directions and speeds; solo and duo; varied actions in feet and legs.

Large ball among four in half of area

With one large ball among four, the eventual game invented will probably have 2 v 2, or 1 v 3; will be played in half of the group's area; and will need one main rule and a scoring system.

Year 2

Lesson Plan 11 • 30 minutes
July

Emphasis on: *(a) planning and performing safely a range of simple actions and linked movements in response to given tasks; (b) demonstrating improvements, generally, in performances that are accurate, consistent and look 'easy'; (c) reflecting competently in pointing out key features and expressing pleasure after observing a performance.*

Warm-up and Footwork Practices
5 minutes

1   Jog easily, 'coasting' along at a speed which you think you can maintain almost as easily as quick walking. In your jogging, arms and heels are lower than in stylish or fast running. Can you 'feel' this rhythm which you find easy to continue?

2   Cross-court relays. Partners stand, side by side, down the middle of the area. On 'Go!' one partner sprints to touch his or her nearer side line, then sprints back to touch partner's outstretched hand. Second partner sprints to own, nearer side line, then back to touch first partner's hand. This continues until the pair have made the number of touches asked for, when the teacher calls out the results.

Skills Practices: with a small ball and bat
5 minutes

Partner practices

1   Batting partner, strike the ball from one hand, high, to give partner an easy catch. Catcher, roll the ball back to your partner. Have six goes then change.

2   Batting partner, strike ball along ground to give partner fielding practice. Fielder, send ball back to batter with one bounce for an easy, one-handed catch. Have six goes and then change.

3   French cricket. Bowler aims ball to hit partner on the leg below knee height, from about 2 metres away, slowly and gently. Batter guards legs with bat held low and turns ball away. Fielder next throws from where he or she picked up the ball. (Game is kept contained by insisting on gentle aiming and hitting.) Change when bowler hits legs of batter.

Group Practices
20 minutes

Long rope in groups of four

Two take turns at swinging the rope low from side to side. Skippers try to come in, skip several times, then move away from the still swinging rope.

4 v 4: three-catch rounders

Batting team has one innings each, striking ball to land in the limited area being used. Batters all follow hitter around the diamond of three skittles. Fielders make three catches and shout 'Stop!' Batters score one run for each skittle.

Partners: short tennis; 1 v 1

A competitive game played over a line or rope 'net'. Decide how to serve to start game, and how to score. How many points in a game before changing ends?

Teaching notes and NC guidance
Development over 4 lessons

Warm-up and Footwork Practices

1   Easy jogging has lower arms and heels than normal athletic, good-style running. The steps are shorter and there is a feeling of a continuing rhythm, which the runner should be able to feel: 'Jog; jog; easy; easy. One, two, three, four. One, two, three four.'

2   In cross-court relays, emphasise that they touch just over the line, each time, with a foot. Also, they must wait to be touched by the incoming partner. (The over-competitive touch short of the line, and go before being touched.) A crouched, sprint-start position by the second runner gets him or her off to a more explosive start.

Skills Practices: with a small bat and ball

Partner practices

1   Ball is struck from hand as in a table-tennis service. Striker should be side-on to receiving partner. 3 metres apart is an easy distance and sufficient for receiver to see ball's speed and flight, and react. 'Keep your best team score of good hits and catches out of 12.'

2   Batter tries to send the ball along ground, without bouncing, for partner to field with both hands and body behind ball. Hands are spread wide with fingers down towards ground, and small fingers can be crossed to 'make a floor for the basket made by the hands'.

3   In French cricket, make it a main rule that the ball stays in the limited area the pair is using. In other words, 'No big hits!' Bowler is enouraged to bowl underarm at a good length, to land ball about half a metre in front of the batter's legs, which are the target. Batter plays a purely defensive stroke to push the ball away 2 or 3 metres to what is the next bowling position.

Group Practices

Long rope in groups of four

In long-rope skipping in fours where two swing and two skip, the rope swingers only swing the rope from side to side, if the skippers are learners. With more expert performers the rope is swung in a complete circle. Both learners and experts move in to skip as the rope swings away from them (i.e. in from left as rope swings up to right). They leave rope one way as it swings the other (i.e. out to left as rope moves to right).

4 v 4: three-catch rounders

In 4-against-4 rounders, the main rule is that the ball must not leave the area allocated. When each one of batting team has had one hit, the teams change over. The three catches of the fielding team must involve three different players. Bowler is asked to bowl underarm to let ball bounce about 1 metre in front of the batter. A bat or a hand can be used for the striking to enable easy hitting.

Partners: short tennis; 1 v 1

The competitive, 1-against-1 short tennis over a long, low rope 'net' can be better contained if chalk marks are made at the sides of each little 'court'. The easiest serve is to drop the ball to make it bounce straight up to be hit at about mid-chest height. Encourage pupils to stand 'side-on' to their opponents, with the chest facing to one side, not towards the opponent.